Adapted Adventure Activities

A Rehabilitation Model for Adventure Programming and Group Initiatives

Wendy Ellmo

Jill Graser

This edition has been printed on recycled paper.

KENDALL/HUNT PUBLISHING COMPANY
4050 Westmark Drive Dubuque, Iowa 52002

ISBN 0-7872-0334-3

Printed in the United States of America

10 9 8 7 6 5 4 3 2 1

Adapted Adventure Activities

Wendy Ellmo
Jill Graser

Illustrations by
Glen A. Schofield

Photographs by
Dave DiPaolo

Dedication

To Frank and Stanley
for their unconditional support, for respecting our work,
but most of all for respecting us.

To Ron and Henrietta Schofield
and Henry and Jeanette Karaman
for raising us to believe in ourselves.

And to our clients,
who make it easy to keep the Adventure alive.

Acknowledgments

Our deepest gratitude to Elizabeth McElwain, CTRS, without whom Initiative Group would not even have been a thought at the Center for Head Injuries. Liz went off to some place called Project Adventure for a workshop about five years ago. She came back, barely able to sit still, rambling on and on about "this place" she went to. Somewhat intrigued, but mostly just to quiet her down, Wendy sat and listened. Several meetings later, Initiative Group began to emerge. She was the uninhibited spirit in the group who was able to convince her co-leader to walk down the hallway (past the clinical director's office!) carrying hoola hoops and water balloons. It just didn't seem to look therapeutic enough. Five years later, we know better. Liz was responsible, in whole or in part, for many of the initial activities, including *Blind Spear Fishing* and *Walkie Talkie Towers,* just to name a couple. She was greatly missed when she left three years ago to pursue other opportunities in California. Liz, for Initiative Group and for being a good friend, we thank you.

Thanks also to Dave DiPaolo, M. Ed., for taking the photographs for the book. He gave up many lunch times and free hours to take photos and pick up and drop off film. Dave, we cherish your humor, creative spirit and friendship.

Glen Schofield — thank you for the great illustrations. Glen, who works professionally as an illustrator and art director, again answered the call to do "just one more" drawing for a family member. Your talent inspires us.

Thank you to Tom Zierk, Publications Director at Project Adventure, for his helpful insights and suggestions. Thank you also for being our advocate at PA and for believing in this project.

Thanks to Mark Murray for leading us at our first PA workshop and showing us first-hand what the Adventure is all about. Thank you also for your suggestions on the manuscript and for making sure that we represented PA's concepts and goals correctly.

Thank you to Barbara Surhoff, B.S., P.T., for her guidance in all of the physical therapy issues and for editing those portions of the manuscript.

And finally, thank you to Keith Cicerone, Ph.D., Clinical Director at the Center for Head injuries and the entire staff at *Cog* for creating an atmosphere where Initiative Group could thrive.

Wendy and Jill
January, 1994

Contents

Appendices

Introduction

We wrote *Adapted Adventure Activities* to share the benefits and fun of Adventure Programming with other professionals working in rehabilitation. We were thrilled when we first learned of Project Adventure and were eager to try the activities with our brain injured clients. We used some activities for a couple of weeks and then ran out of suitable ones because of our clients' decreased cognition, communication and physical abilities. Undaunted, we began creating our own! *Adapted Adventure Activities* will introduce you to Adventure Programming, show you how to make it work for rehabilitation populations, and provide you with many of our favorite activities.

The first section of the book helps you to build a foundation and a context for the activities that follow in the second section. Chapter 1 provides you with the theory behind Project Adventure, a non-profit organization with offices scattered around the world, and upon which our program, Initiative Group, is based. Chapter 2 shows how we have adapted Project Adventure's practices to meet our needs within a therapeutic setting. Chapter 3 discusses what types of populations may benefit from Initiative Group and what therapeutic disciplines might use it. This chapter also details ways of modifying activities so that they will work for your unique population. Chapter 4 highlights some logistical ideas that have made the day-to-day running of Initiative Group much simpler for us. We think you'll find them helpful.

The second section is filled with activities for you to try. They are primarily a collection of Initiatives — activities designed to address predominantly problem solving and other cognitive skills. All of them require group cooperation and communication to ensure their success. Where appropriate, we included potential modifications and variations for you to try. There is also information about how to process the experience with your group to make it a more effective learning experience. The activities are presented alphabetically to make finding a particular one easy.

Appendices I, II, III and IV break down the activities by group size, group format (group, pairs and group versus group) and type of action (table top versus up and moving). These appendices are helpful when you know the size of your group, the format you would like to use or the physical activity level you want but don't have a particular activity in mind. The final appendix, V, lists activities from other sources that we particularly like for our brain injured clients or ones that we believe would be appropriate for special populations. This appendix will help you to enlarge your adventure base.

After playing around unsuccessfully with constantly writing "he or she" and "he/she" when referring to our clients, we eventually decided to go simply with "he". This was a tough decision for two pretty independent females! We reasoned that since, statistically, more men than women are involved in accidents resulting in traumatic brain injuries, that meant that, statistically at least, most of our clients were men. Therefore, we decided to go with the majority and stick with the masculine pronoun. We hope that this decision does not offend anyone. If it does, please consider the he's, his' and him's to be genderless and universal. Enough said.

Any clients' names used are fictitious.

We hope that *Adapted Adventure Activities* will change the way you think about group therapy — or at least expand it — and that it will encourage more creativity in your treatment planning. Good luck and have fun!

Section One

Have you ever pushed yourself to the limit? Have you ever experienced the rush of nervous energy and excitement of anticipation before tackling a physical, intellectual or emotional challenge? How about the feeling of pride and satisfaction — and the self-confidence — after completing that challenge?

Positive changes in self-confidence and overall self-image have been shown to be positively correlated with a high degree of healthy risk taking. Are you a risk taker? What is healthy risk taking? It depends on each individual's perception of what type of risk he or she grows from. It depends on what type of experience, when completed, leaves you with a sense of self-confidence and pride. We have all experienced this at some time and have observed others in this stage. It is recognized by a highly held head, upright posture, confident stride, and slightly concealed smile which says, "*I went for it and I am proud!*"

But ...how often do we see that telling smile on the faces of our rehabilitation clients? More often, what we see lack is of confidence, frustration and disappointment. Section One will give you the foundation you need to begin changing those negative self-images, feelings and abilities into positive ones.

In Section One you will find:

- A brief history and philosophy of the models our group was based on and of Adventure Based Counseling (Chapter One);
- A complete explanation of how Initiative Group was adapted to fit the complex needs of rehabilitation populations (Chapter Two);
- What populations can benefit from using this program (Chapter Three);
- Guidelines for adapting any activity to fit the special needs of your population (Chapter Three) and;
- Practical considerations for starting your own Initiative Group (Chapter Four).

Chapter One

The Foundations For Initiative Group

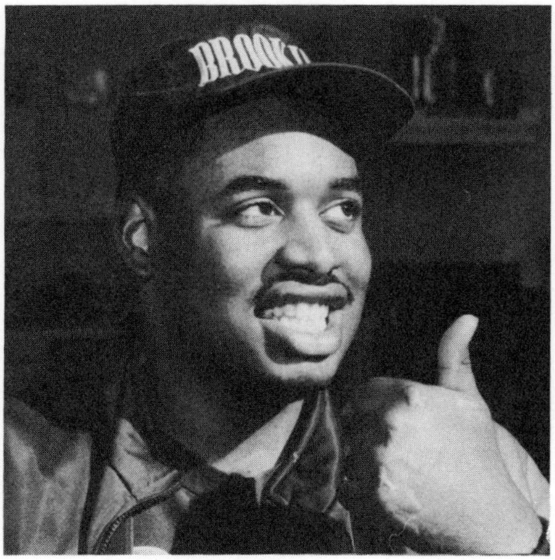

All too often, unfortunately, the rehabilitation process focuses on deficits, leaving clients questioning their abilities and feeling isolated and incompetent. Initiative Group, at the Center for Head Injuries, was developed to reverse this, to help people go through rehabilitation and come out once again feeling like whole individuals, with a sense of confidence and self-worth. Initiative Group structures adventure based activities to provide the opportunity for successful group experiences, helping clients to break the string of failure experiences, and thus facilitate further growth. The clients in Initiative Group learn experientially by being exposed to a variety of new situations. The group provides a motivating and non-threatening environment where members can develop their group interaction, cognitive, physical, emotional, communicative and other skills.

Adventure based activities are what make Initiative Group unique to traditional rehabilitation approaches. We have found that the elements of risk and fun inherent in each activity successfully engage clients in the tasks. Traditional rehabilitation methods tend to have a major focus on paper and pencil tasks and few real-life interactions. Clients find the experiential learning process extremely effective in developing functional life skills and improving carryover and generalization for managing their lives outside of the group.

These three elements:

1. ability to engage clients
2. emphasis on functional skills
3. ease of generalization

are necessary to consider when treatment planning for *all* rehabilitation populations. Also important when the busy professional selects treatment tasks, is whether those tasks are easily adaptable to different types and levels of clients. The Initiative Group tasks successfully meet all of these requirements.

Project Adventure and Adventure Based Counseling

Our group rehabilitation model, Initiative Group, is based on the concepts and activities of Project Adventure, whose philosophy holds that people are usually more capable (mentally, emotionally and physically) than they perceive themselves to be. Project Adventure games and activities give people opportunities to challenge themselves and to take risks within the supportive atmosphere of the group. To PA, *Adventure* means any new experience that elicits excitement. They use non-competitive games, group problem-solving Initiatives, and ropes course events to create that excitement and achieve their goals of facilitating personal learning and growth.

The use of adventure/risk activities to promote experiential learning is not a new concept. PA is based on the theories of the Outward Bound wilderness training program originated in England by Dr. Kurt Hahn. The Outward Bound program primarily utilized wilderness survival experiences, which made this method of instruction inaccessible to most schools. Jerry Pieh, a Massachusetts high school principal, and his staff started PA by adapting the successful Outward Bound strategies to fit a typical school setting. Pieh's vision was for this teaching and learning method to become an integral part of standard high school curriculum.

Pieh incorporated two major modifications into this new method of Adventure Programming:

- Activities were changed to be more accessible by decreasing intensity, cost and duration through the use of rope courses, Initiatives and games.
- Structure was increased throughout each activity.

Probably the most well-known portions to come out of Pieh's original program are the Initiatives and the challenge ropes course. Initiatives are problems that are presented by the instructor to be solved by the group, and are structured to promote group cooperation, trust and communication. A ropes course consists of high and low elements that are built outside in trees or inside in a gym. They are designed to facilitate both individual challenge and group cooperation.

Out of Adventure Programming grew Adventure Based Counseling (ABC). ABC groups involve special identified populations — troubled youths and psychological counseling groups, for example. For ABC groups, the emphasis is less on the actual activity and more on what is learned *from* the activity. Participants are helped to relate the learning to their daily lives and interactions with others.

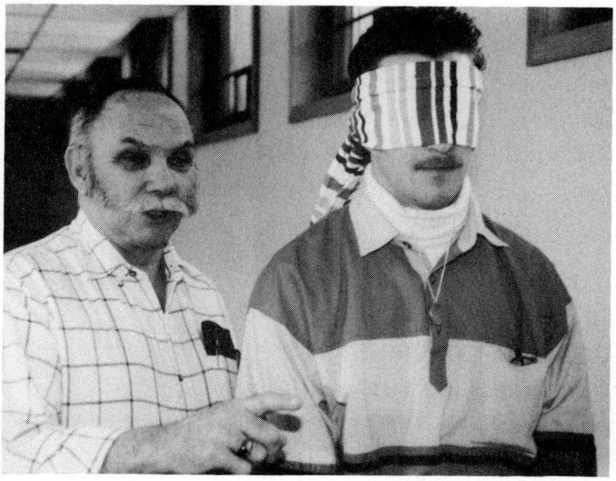

The main goal of both Adventure Programming and ABC is to *improve the self-concept* of its participants. Carl Rogers defined self-concept as the way "an individual perceives himself in relation to the world around him" (*Islands of Healing*, Schoel, Prouty & Radcliffe, 1989). It is your image of who you are and what you value in yourself and in your relationships with others. The primary cause of a negative self-concept appears to be a series of failure experiences that set the stage for a lack of confidence in new tasks, relationships and decision-making.

PA believes that a positive self-concept can be developed through an improved sense of *trust* and *competence*. Adventure based activities successfully access these two areas by providing opportunities for participants to experience the feelings of trust and success in a group. These experiences can then be shared and validated through the group.

Adventure Based Programming — Six Key Elements

Adventure programming involves more than simply choosing an activity to develop a certain skill. It requires planning and organization on the part of the group leaders to create an atmosphere of learning and interaction. Six key elements have been identified by PA to meet this goal.

1. Trust Building
2. Goal Setting
3. Challenge/Stress
4. Ah Ha! Experiences
5. Humor/Fun
6. Problem Solving

Trust Building

Activities that develop trust are an important component of the Adventure Based Counseling (ABC) process. Trust is developed through a series of physical trust-building activities, which are *required* of all participants. Group members learn that they can trust the group and rely on others to be there. From these beginnings of physical trust, the activities move to more complex psycho-social interaction trust issues. Further on, participants learn to risk appearing foolish, failing or being vulnerable — all within the supportive and non-threatening atmosphere of the group. The goal of the trust activities is to develop group cohesion and a sense of teamwork.

Goal Setting

Studies show that people experience greater psychological success if they set and define their own realistic yet challenging goals. The more active group members are in their own goal setting, the more vested they are in the group process because they can see how it relates to themselves. Goal setting helps keep the individual focused and helps make the transfer of progress to other environments easier.

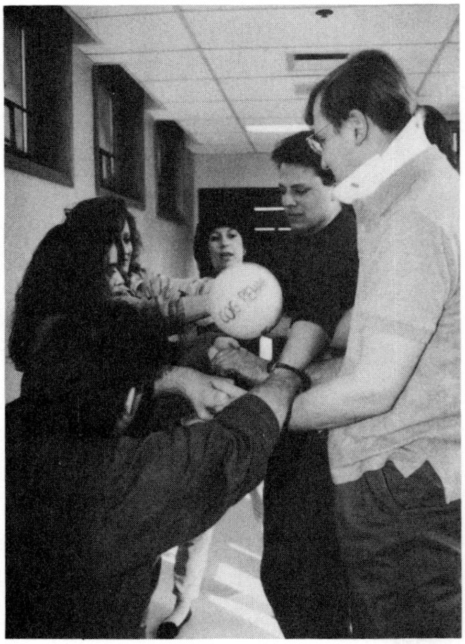

Challenge/Stress

Adventure experiences must involve perceived risks and tasks that are physically and/or intellectually demanding but achievable. PA removes activities from the thrill seeking and focuses on self-improvement by setting individual and group goals. Under these challenging circumstances, group members experience a strong feeling of success and accomplishment once the task is completed and their goal is met. PA teaches how to deal with stress effectively by approaching it with an attitude that will produce a balanced or positive stress response. It emphasizes anticipation and a *Go for it — Positively* attitude.

Ah Ha! Experience

An Ah Ha! experience is a culmination point where everything comes together and the individual learns some truth about himself or his relationship within the group. It may be, for example, when someone feels some measure of success or self-pride because she supported another person through a stressful experience. This feeling of pride may be conscious or unconscious. The Ah Ha! experience can be planned or spontaneous.

Humor/Fun

Challenged populations have a harder time laughing. PA uses the curing power of laughter as an intrinsic stress-fighting mechanism to help restore physical and mental balance. Group leaders may present an activity with humor, the activity itself may be based on a funny story, or individual goals may be to act foolish, let go and laugh.

Problem Solving

The Adventure Based Counseling model continually puts group members in situations where they must solve problems by working together as a group. Participants are presented with a problem, told their parameters, and asked to solve it in the best way possible. They are shown by necessity the need for good problem-solving skills and are able to process both positive and negative experiences within a supportive, safe environment. Motivation and persistence are encouraged. Overt identification of specific problem-solving skills and attitudes during processing time helps to transfer them to daily life.

The Full Value Contract

One of Project Adventure's most valuable and important concepts is called the Full Value Contract (FVC). It is founded in the belief that every individual group member and the group itself have value, and it incorporates the behavior guidelines for the group. In becoming a member of Initiative Group, each person agrees to abide by this contract.

According to *Islands of Healing*, the Full Value Contract engenders three main ideas:

1. Agreement to work together as a group and to work toward individual and group goals;
2. Agreement to adhere to certain safety and group behavior guidelines;
3. Agreement to give and receive feedback, both positive and negative, and to work toward changing behavior when it is appropriate (pg. 95).

The Full Value Contract provides a way of setting limits for the group in a positive way. Everyone agrees to give full effort and to value the group. Each member agrees to speak up when they see something unsafe happening. Each group member agrees to let others know when they are doing something that violates their personal goal or a group goal. They also commit to accept feedback from each other. Each individual agrees to self-monitor — to make it known when they themselves have violated a trust, a goal or a rule. It is critical, though, that group leaders monitor the intensity of the confronting and know how much feedback the group can handle at any time.

Implicit in this agreement is that it *will* be broken. There will be times when someone does not give his or her all or does not feel safe enough confronting another person. This is especially likely to happen when a group is new or a member is new. New clients will need time to develop trust and to feel comfortable being honest and open with the other members. That is okay, because, in the spirit of the Adventure Wave, there is always another chance to come back and try it again. The Adventure Wave refers to the activity sequence discussed below — the brief, activity and debrief. This sequence is a part of every group session. The cycle repeats itself over and over again, just like waves, where there is always another activity behind the one you can see. It gives group members the comforting feeling that they can decline a challenge one day, because there will be another opportunity to try again in the future.

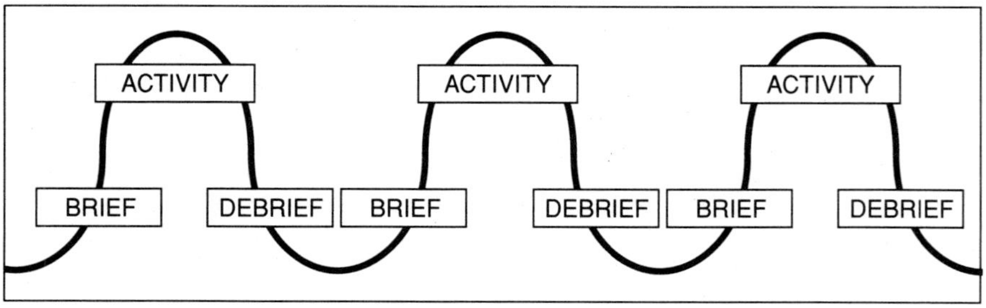

An immediate feedback system is essential for the group to be effective. This requires a commitment from all group members to be open and honest with themselves as well as other group members. The use of the FVC as the tool to reinforce this process has proven to be very effective.

The Full Value Contract and goal setting are essential to the Adventure Based Counseling process. The FVC helps members stay focused on their own goals and to remember that others have goals as well. They build an immediate feedback system and commitment to self and others into the program.

Activity Sequence — Brief, Activity, Debrief

Each PA session is divided into three important, sequenced, phases. These phases incorporate active processing into the activity sessions, serving to distinguish this model from skill development and wilderness training programs. The three phases are called *Brief, Activity* and *Debrief.*

Brief

Briefing is initiated by the group leaders, who begin by framing the experience or focusing group members on what is to come. The leaders provide directions for the activity and also give any rules or restrictions and safety guidelines. The group members are then involved by setting their own goals for the activity. (Refer to *Islands of Healing,* pg. 103, for guidelines on how to set effective goals.) During the brief, the leaders may remind the group of their commitment to adhere to the Full Value Contract — to do their best to value themselves and others and to provide feedback when the contract is violated. The leader also challenges group members to challenge themselves while doing the activity. The members may raise concerns based on past events that are relevant to the new task. Those concerns are discussed and plans are made for a fresh start.

Activity

The activities are the means for experiential learning. They are carefully chosen by the group leaders according to the level of their group. The leaders remain active group members, challenging the group to push beyond their perceived physical and emotional capabilities, but not providing information about how to solve the problem. The leaders remain ready to intervene to refocus the group, to ensure that safety guidelines are adhered to, or to help the clients address an issue arising within the group. Leaders act as models for

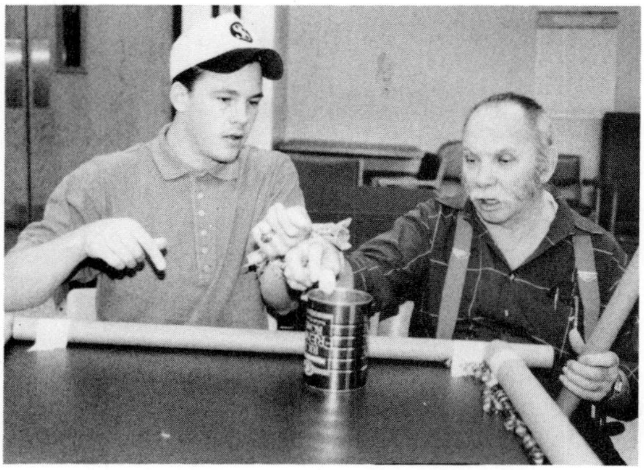

appropriate group behavior. The group must feel that the leaders are with them during an activity even if they are not active participants.

The concept of Challenge By Choice (*Islands of Healing,* pg. 131) is always operating, meaning that all challenges during the activity are taken by choice. No one is ever pressured into doing something that they do not want to do. Challenge By Choice is a very important concept in all Adventure Based programming. It allows the participant to try to do something or decide not to and to be supported regardless of the decision. It places more importance on the attempt rather than on the actual outcome. Because of the Adventure Wave concept, the individual knows that if he elects not to take the challenge today, there will always be an opportunity to take it again in the future.

Debrief

Debriefing is the process of talking about the adventure experience. Leaders must avoid the temptation to let the activity stand on its own. Just because some growth or learning was obvious to them, they must never assume that the group was aware of it as well. Group leaders must be prepared to help the group deal with potentially sensitive issues of resistance and conflict. They must be confident in their ability to lead the group through it. The debrief should not be a lecture by the leaders. Instead, the leaders should guide the participants through raising and addressing issues on their own in the positive spirit of the Full Value Contract. Everyone is encouraged to participate but even here, during the debrief, the idea of Challenge by Choice operates.

The debrief phase uses three basic questions to ease the group into discussing the experience:

1. What
2. So What
3. Now What

First, members are asked ***What*** happened? They begin with the facts. They discuss the substance of the group interaction and what happened to the individuals. This question then leads into the remainder of the processing stage.

The next question asked is ***So What***? "What difference did it make?" Group members should be encouraged to abstract and generalize from the experience. They are also asked to evaluate their performance with respect to their group and individual goals and to give others feedback on their performance.

Next, they are challenged with ***Now What***? This involves deciding how to apply what they have learned to the next session. They are asked to generalize what implications this activity might have on real life and how the skills they used might be important in their daily lives. Sessions are ended with hopes for better things to come and with the positive expectation that these skills will be used outside of the session and will help the individual be more successful. The debrief is utilized not only at the end of an activity, but at any time the leaders feel it is necessary to reflect more deeply and overtly on what is happening.

Conclusion

We have provided a brief overview of Project Adventure's philosophy because it is very important to incorporate these theories into treatment planning. The activities in this book all have the potential for excellent cognitive, physical, communicative and emotional skill development, but it is the way in which they are implemented and processed that will determine their effectiveness for your clients.

For a more complete discussion of PA's background and philosophy, read *Islands of Healing: A Guide to Adventure Based Counseling* by Jim Schoel, Dick Prouty and Paul Radcliffe (Project Adventure, Inc., 1989).

For more information on how to include disabled individuals in a traditional Adventure program, read *Bridges to Accessibility: A Primer for Including Persons with Disabilities in Adventure Curricula* by Mark D. Havens (Project Adventure, Inc., 1992).

For information on Adventure Based Counseling workshops, contact Project Adventure.

Chapter Two

The Rehabilitation Model: Adapting Adventure Based Counseling For Use In Clinical Settings

When Initiative Group first started, it wasn't Initiative Group at all. It was called *Speech Group*. Not very imaginative, huh? It was supposed to address a wide range of communication skills, especially pragmatics or social skills. We spent a lot of time sitting around a table, discussing appropriate behavior and role playing various situations.

There was one specific day when things went particularly well. We had been role playing difficult situations that might occur in the community — arguments with bank tellers, that kind of thing. One of the clients, Michelle, had done surprisingly well. She had asserted herself and maintained her cool despite several mistakes made by Joe, our fictitious department store clerk. Michelle was the one in the unit who, when you came out of a treatment session with her, whoever had her next would come running up to you demanding to know what kind of mood she was in. You knew that if Michelle was having a bad day, you were in for it. Most of Michelle's days were bad. So on this day we felt as if we had made a real breakthrough, and we were feeling pretty good. That is, until

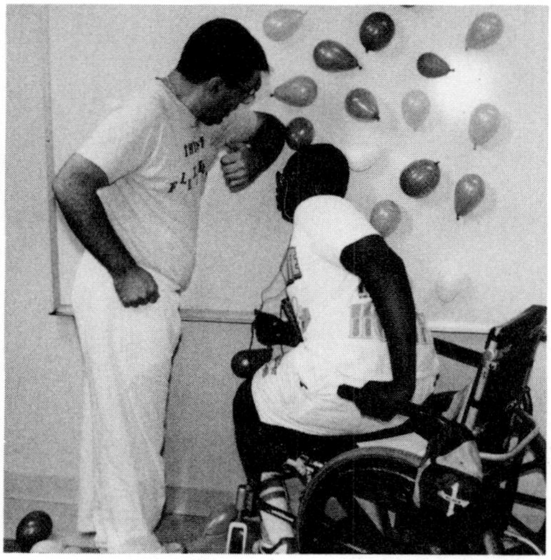

we followed the group out of the room after the session. Joe looked at Michelle, apparently the wrong way, and she shouted, "What the @#)*! are you looking at!"

We knew we had to rethink things.

It was around this time that Liz McElwain, who co-led the group, went to a workshop at Project Adventure to learn about Adventure Based Counseling. Liz came back very excited and anxious to share what she had learned. We liked the whole concept and saw the obvious benefits: a place where our clients could have fun and increase their self-esteem, yet still work on their other physical, cognitive and communicative goal areas. We were excited. We began to see a way of working on traditional rehabilitation goals, but doing it in a more nontraditional way. A way that focused less on what a person could *not* do and more on what they *could.*

How Initiative Group Came to Be

After a little thought and some experimentation with PA activities, we began to see some drawbacks. We work with outpatient and residential moderately to mildly brain injured clients for the JFK-Johnson Rehabilitation Institute, a non-profit facility. Given our population, many of the activities were too physically based, too cognitively challenging, or did not meet the goals we were trying to achieve. Also, because our clients' injuries are relatively recent, they are not yet even comfortable with less risky activities — like walking down a hallway in a new leg brace, maneuvering around in a tight space in a wheelchair, or riding in a car with a vestibular problem. A lot of other activities were out because of the number of participants needed. In rehabilitation, groups tend to be small, typically between three and eight people. There were some Initiatives that we were able to use as is and others that were perfect after a bit of modification. We also found that we needed to make some changes to the briefing and debriefing stages.

What was left when all the dust settled was Initiative Group. We believe that Initiative Group can be further fine-tuned to work with most other special needs populations (see Chapter Three for *Who Can Use Initiative Group* and more on modifying activities).

What Initiative Group is able to do is provide a motivating and non-threatening environment in which clients can practice their compensatory strategies. Our feedback to the clients is probably more positive than in other groups where increasing clients' awareness of their deficits may also be a primary goal. The message that we are trying to give them is, "Yes, you can be successful." It is believed that a negative self-concept is developed through a succession of failure experiences. The very nature of rehab is that most of our clients come to us with some awareness problems (at least in brain injury rehabilitation), so a major part of our day is spent constantly showing them that they are different.

Another portion of our clients know that they have deficits but are reluctant to use their compensatory strategies because of what people might say or because it "feels different" than before. Rehabilitation often leaves clients feeling isolated and incompetent. What we are saying to them in Initiative Group is, "WOW! You used that strategy and you were successful," or, when the group fails, we process the failure, find out why, and hold it out as a goal to be accomplished next time. The message here is, "Well, we did not do it this time, but there is always next time." By creating a goal from their failure, we are helping the clients to fail in a positive way. Or, as PA trainer Ken Demas puts it, we are allowing them to *fail forward.* We are helping them to turn a failure into a learning experience, turning failure into opportunity. Now that we know what to do, we will come back and try it again. This is how we use the Adventure Wave. There is always another activity coming along behind this one; there is always another chance to succeed. What we are allowing them to do is feel competent. We are breaking the string of failure experiences and giving our clients a sense of self so they can take risks in order to grow further.

Components of Initiative Group

For our clients, *risk* might simply mean sharing ideas despite expressive language problems or using a cane to walk down the aisle at a wedding. It does not have to mean risk in the typical life-threatening sense. Risk is anything that is perceived by individuals as something challenging that, once attempted, provides an opportunity to grow.

Group Formation

Group formation is a constant issue in our minds because our members are always changing. Presently, we are running Initiative Group as a cognitive/communication group. However, physical and counseling goals are often incorporated. The criteria for admission into the group are kept very broad. The flexible nature of the group allows for it to work even with a heterogeneous group. And can it get heterogeneous! In fact, diversity seems to be the rule rather than the exception. At times, our groups have had people in them from their teens to their seventies, from artists to engineers, from Peru to Portugal; people with traumatically induced brain injuries to anoxia, strokes or arteriovenous malformations. Most of the time we are pleasantly surprised with how well things go. We do spend a lot of time initially thinking about what might go wrong or be difficult and then we attempt to work around it (see Chapter Three on *Modifying Activities*).

Our admission criteria are broad. We will accept anyone into the group who:

- has receptive and/or expressive communication problems
- has difficulty with pragmatics (social skills)
- is not confident with their communication skills (low self-esteem) or
- has cognitive deficits including: problem solving, initiation, attention, concentration, planning, etc.

Notice that we have no physical restrictions or criteria. We will adapt our activities to fit the physical level(s) of the group. The admission criteria for your group will obviously reflect your own population and particular discipline.

Sequencing

Activity sequencing is a very important consideration in ABC. The first step in planning a sequence of activities (or Adventure Wave Plan) for your group is to define a set of goals and objectives for the group. These are the general and specific outcomes that you hope the group will achieve.

With these goals and objectives in place and clearly defined, you are ready to begin selecting activities to help the group meet them. PA divides activities into seven main categories, while recognizing that there can be significant overlap between the areas. These categories are:

Ice Breaker/Acquaintance
To provide opportunities for group members to get to know each other and to begin feeling comfortable with each other through activities, Initiatives and games that are primarily fun, non-threatening and group-based.

De-Inhibitizer
To provide a setting wherein group participants are able to take some risks as well as make improvement in commitment and a willingness to appear inept in front of others.

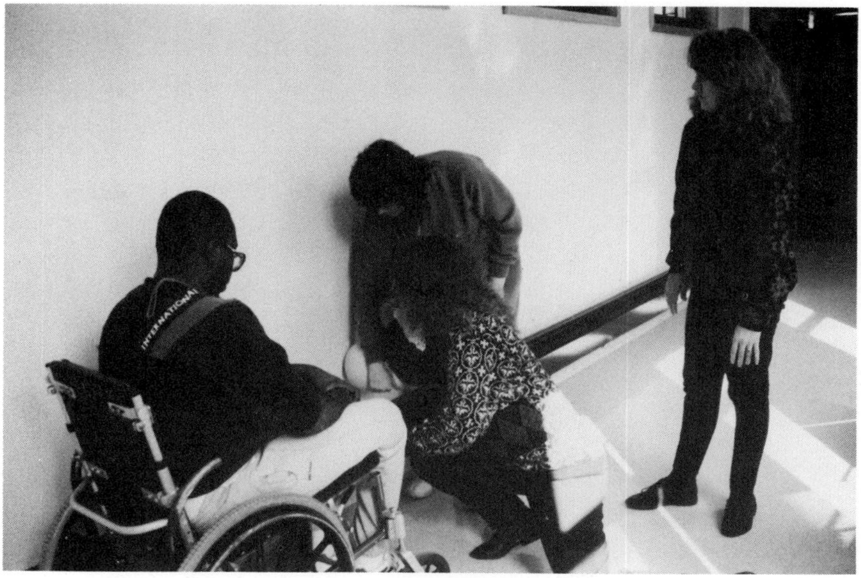

Trust and Empathy
To provide an opportunity for group members to trust their physical and emotional safety with others by attempting a graduated series of activities that involve taking some physical and/or emotional risks.

Communication
To provide an opportunity for group members to enhance their ability and skill to communicate thoughts, feelings and behaviors more appropriately through activities which emphasize listening, verbal and physical skills in the group decision-making process.

Decision-Making/Problem-Solving
To provide an opportunity for group members to effectively communicate, cooperate and compromise with each other through trial-and-error participation in a graduated series of problem-solving activities which range from the more simply solved to the more complex.

Social Responsibility
To provide a setting wherein group participants can build upon previous gains in areas of acquaintance, trust, communications and decision-making, to develop skill in assessing and working effectively with the strengths and weaknesses of individuals in a group.

Personal Responsibility
To provide activities and Initiatives of a somewhat more individualistic nature which challenge participants to develop persistence and resistance to frustration in attempting to reach a desired goal. (*Islands of Healing*, pg. 280)

The categories are not to be interpreted as being hierarchical, and they should be moved between flexibly as needed. The first three categories, though, often help to build a firm foundation within the group for the bigger challenges to come. There is also no set amount of time for groups to spend doing each type of activity. Groups should move at their own pace.

The GRABBS Modality Check List is helpful to use in choosing activities:

Goals—How does the activity relate to the group and individual goals that have been set?

Readiness—This regards levels of instruction (skills) and safety capabilities. Is the group ready to do the activity? Will they endanger themselves and others? Do they have the ability to attempt or complete? What will you have to do to change the event to compensate for lack of readiness?

Affect—What is the feeling of the group? What kinds of sensations are they having? What is the level of empathy or caring in the group?

Behavior—How is the group acting? Are they resistive? Disruptive? Agreeable? Are they more self involved, or group involved? Are there any interactions that are affecting the group, both positive and negative? How cooperative are they?

Body—What kind of physical shape are they in? How tired are they? Do they substance abuse? Are they on medication? How do they see their own bodies?

Stage—Which developmental stage is the group at? Groups will go through all levels of functioning. Having a schema to describe these levels will provide you with another means of assessment. (*Islands of Healing*, pg. 80)

The GRABBS Check List is best used in conjunction with Chapter Three of this book. Chapter Three will help you to tailor the activity you have chosen to best fit the specific and unique needs of your rehabilitation group. Be prepared to adjust your Adventure Wave Plan to meet the needs of your group. Again, see Chapter Four of *Islands of Healing* for a more in-depth look at developing and adjusting an Adventure Wave Plan.

In a clinical setting, we do not always have the ability to move through the sequence in the way we would like. Clients are admitted to the group whenever their treatment team decides it is appropriate, regardless of where the group is at. Clients are also discharged at various times depending on issues like clinical appropriateness, scheduling conflicts and funding problems. So, people always seem to be coming and going in Initiative Group. We need to be sensitive to sequencing issues, but we cannot always move through the sequence in an ideal way. Which activity we decide to do on a day when a new client is admitted to the group depends on a number of factors, including:

- How much we know about the client's interaction style, cognition and communication;
- Where the group is at. Are they accepting of new people? Are they comfortable with themselves as a group?
- How well the new client knows the other group members from other groups or the lunch room.

We do not place a lot of expectations on new group members for their first couple of times in group. We allow them to step back and just get comfortable with how the group operates. We increase expectations and feedback after that. The most common problem we encounter by not being able to move through a proper sequencing cycle is members not feeling comfortable touching each other during the physical activities and not being completely supportive of each other during cognitively and communicatively intense activities. When these problems arise we spend extra time processing them during the debrief and brainstorming potential solutions with the group for next time.

Another major issue we encounter with sequencing is that our clients do not place much value on the ice breaker, de-inhibitizer and trust activities. Most of our clients are with us to work and get better and are not interested in doing anything where they cannot see the direct benefit in their lives. They don't see that going through these categories will help them to work better with the group and ultimately learn more about themselves and others. Their own personal goal has nothing to do with working better with this group or learning about anyone else.

So, we often need to skip great activities (depending on the group makeup) that don't have an overt cognitive or communication emphasis. Physically oriented groups may not experience the same problems because they can highlight several physical goals while also working on trust issues. We might instead use something like the *TP Shuffle* (*Silver Bullets*, pg. 110), which does overtly involve communication and problem solving but also brings in trust and touching issues. The cognitive and linguistic demands in the *TP Shuffle* are typically manageable for beginning groups.

PREDICTION/EVALUATION CHECKLIST

Date:____________

Group Goals	Predict Yes	Predict No	Evaluate Yes	Evaluate No
1. I will support other group members				
2. I will give feedback to others				
3. I will speak up when a rule is broken				

Personal Goals	Predict Yes	Predict No	Evaluate Yes	Evaluate No
1.				
2.				
3.				
4.				

Summary:

Think about your setting and the people you work with to begin to anticipate some of the sequencing dilemmas that might surface. Sequencing needs to be a primary consideration but it may not always be ideal given the unique qualities of rehabilitation populations.

Goals

There are three group goals that everyone works on and two to four personal goals that are different for each person (See Prediction Evaluation Checklist, page 20). The group goals reflect the Full Value Contract. The individual goals are tailored to each client's specific deficits. If one of the leaders is not the primary therapist on a specific case, we consult with that therapist to develop that client's personal goals. And, depending on the primary reason for admission into the group, we might also consult with the counselor, therapeutic recreation specialist, physical therapist, occupational therapist and neuropsychologist as well. The goals are always shared with and agreed to by the client before they become "official." The physical therapist is consulted before all physically challenging activities for either client restrictions or special needs. The goals are typically in the form of compensatory strategies. For example, "I will ask questions when I do not understand," rather than, "I will improve my auditory comprehension." What this does is provide the clients with a method for achieving their goals and improving their performance. Of course, the goals are modified as appropriate.

Three Main Stages — The Activity Sequence

Like all Adventure Programming groups, each Initiative Group session contains a briefing stage, time when the group performs the activity, and a debriefing stage.

Briefing

During the briefing stage, the activity is explained and members check "Yes" or "No" in the prediction column of their goal sheets for each specific goal. We find that for the head injured, we need these sheets in order to make the briefing process more structured and concrete. Often, one of us will set up a client to be a leader. We will explain the activity to one member ahead of time — maybe in an individual session — so he or she can be responsible for leading the group. Or, we will give the activity name to an old-timer in the group and see if he can remember it or find it in his notes and explain it to the rest of the group. This has been an extremely successful technique for fostering leadership and self-confidence. We have also found it very helpful to brainstorm the possible purposes for the activity right after they have heard the explanation of it. Because our clients generally are concrete thinkers, they tend to look at the surface of the activity and not at the underlying skills required.

Activity

During the second stage, the actual performance of the activity, we do as little cueing as possible. We allow them to fail, feel frustrated and then to work themselves through it. We have found that even when they fail, the group can walk out feeling successful because they worked hard as a team. The only time we will definitely step in is when safety is in question. Almost always, we work with them as part of the team or as an extra body. There is very much a feeling that we are all in this together.

During this stage, a lot of experiential learning takes place. Group members learn by doing. There is less of a worry about generalization to other situations than in other therapy approaches because they are placed in a variety of different situations, many of which are very "real life."

All of the activities that *we* use include some combination of these four elements:

Affect — through trust building, challenge and empathy-provoking experiences

Behavior — or action through physically-based activities

Cognition — through goal setting and problem solving elements

Communication — All of the activities require communication for successful completion. No one member can do it on his own. And if he can, we will impose a rule to force group communication. For example, a rule might be that no one may use both hands. On two-handed tasks, this rule effectively forces clients to talk to one another to get the job done.

Debriefing

During the final stage, debriefing, clients evaluate their actual performance with respect to their goals by checking Yes or No in the *evaluate* column on their goal sheets. This format allows clients to learn first by doing and then to gain insight later during the debriefing process. This is where we go back and compare their

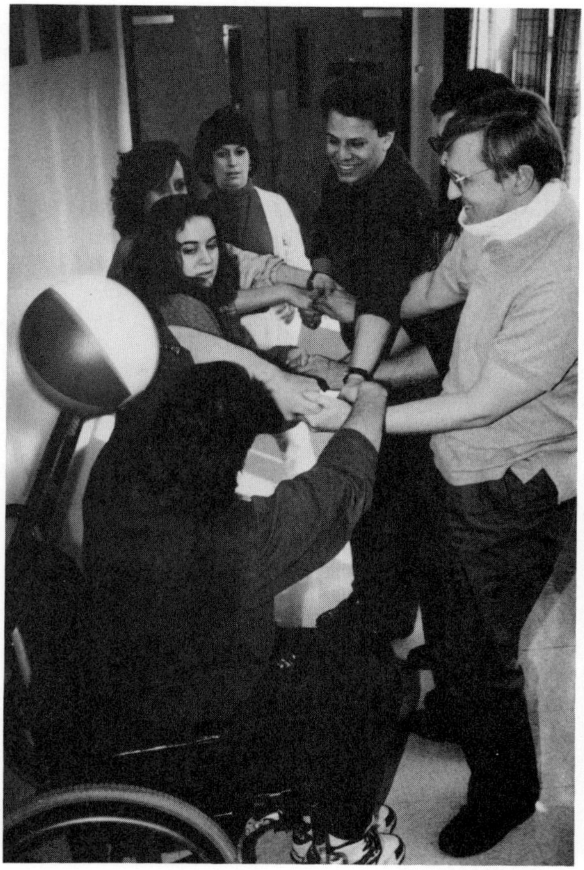

predicted performance with their actual performance. Any discrepancies between the two are discussed to help close the gap between self-perception and reality. So, if someone predicts they are going to do great and they actually had some problems with a particular strategy, they are beginning to see that there may be some residual impairments they could be working on after all. Generally, a pattern that we see is that when clients first come into the group their predictions and evaluations match — they are going to do great! Then, as they are in the group awhile, both start to drop as they become more realistic. Then, after more time, both begin to go up again as they truly improve. These sheets then serve as a way of monitoring changes in their self-awareness. Actually, they do not need to achieve intellectual insight, which is sometimes impossible with significant memory or organic awareness problems. They can still leave the group feeling better and more positive about themselves. We have seen change in goal areas even in clients who did not see the particular area as a problem to be worked on. At some level they incorporated the feedback and experiences and made the necessary changes.

A good debriefing technique we have learned from Project Adventure is the *What, So What, Now What. What* is simply what we did. *So What* is why we did it. We talk about what skills we worked on and make very overt connections to real life. "When might you need these skills? When might you be in a situation like this?" Again, this increases the chances for generalization. *Now What* asks, "Where do we go from here? How can we apply what we learned today to the next activity?" We will often tell the group about the next activity or even continue an activity to a second day, giving them a reason to come back.

During debriefing we focus not just on the outcome, but also on the process. In fact, sometimes very little time is spent on the actual outcome. The emphasis is on "Did you communicate? Did you use your balance or vision strategies? How did you feel while you did this activity? Did you work together as a team? What would you change if you were to do this again?"

The debrief is probably the most important phase with a disabled population. The activity phase, with all of its experiential learning, can be worthless without the debrief to help integrate the experience. Just because you saw wonderful (or terrible!) things taking place during the activity, do not take it for granted that the group saw the same things. Even if they were aware of some of it, take this opportunity to integrate it further.

Videotaping, another debriefing technique, helps our clients compensate for memory deficits and self-monitoring problems, assisting them in accurately assessing their own behavior. We periodically spend a session or two watching videotapes of past sessions. For that day, we structure a discussion — usually based on a problem that had been occurring in recent sessions (see sample videotape sheets). Initially, we focus on teamwork to develop a sense of openness and collaboration within the group. Later, as the clients are more comfortable with each other, the focus typically is shifted to a more direct topic, such as giving and receiving feedback, during which the critical assessment/review of an individual group member's performance is spoken by peers — not therapists. A reminder that we use from time to time during the debrief is that saying, "You did good," is not good enough. You need to say *what* was good. Clients typically enjoy seeing themselves on tape. We have seen some dramatic changes in a couple of members after seeing themselves, because they had no idea they were doing what they saw. The videotapes make the self-evaluation process more concrete.

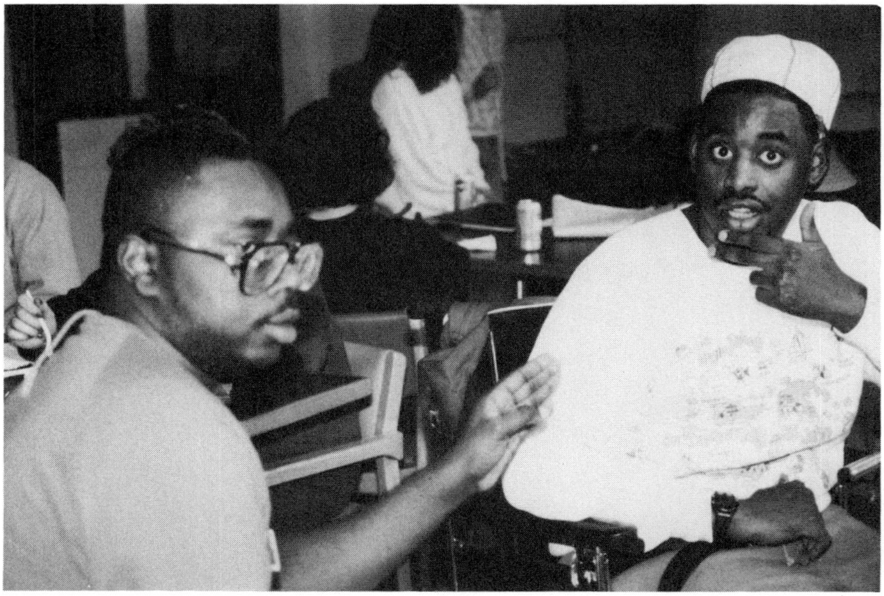

Initiative Group Video Review

Theme: Group Problem Solving

Things to Look For

1. What was the group's approach to solving the problem?
2. Was the problem clearly understood by all members?
3. Did everyone in the group express their opinion when a choice was available?
4. What steps are involved in problem-solving? How are these different in a group as opposed to when you are by yourself?

Theme: Group Interaction Style

Things to Look For

1. Was there a leader?
2. What role did you take?
   a) Were you active?
   b) Were you passive?
   c) Were you sometimes both?
3. Can you think of a specific example of when the entire group cooperated in completing the task?
4. How would you change things in the future to make it work more effectively for the team?

Theme: Group Interaction Style

Positive feedback: Praise given to acknowledge a person's positive actions or statements.

Constructive Criticism: Giving feedback on a person's weakness in a supportive manner.

Negative Feedback: Giving feedback on a person's performance in an aggressive, negative or condescending manner.

Things to Look For:

1. What was the atmosphere of the group — cooperative, active, passive, non-communicative?
2. What type of feedback did you see in this video— positive, constructive, negative?
3. How does this feedback affect the group's interaction style?
4. How do you feel when you or another member receives negative/aggressive feedback?
5. How can you respond to negative feedback to make a positive interaction?

Elements That Make It Work

We have identified 6 key elements that seem to play a major role in making the Initiative Group format and activities successful in terms of client engagement, enjoyment, goal attainment and generalization. They are:

1. Competition
2. Physical Challenge
3. Props/Odd Additions/Humor
4. Moderate Structure
5. Independence
6. Positive Attitude

Competition generates morale, team pride and self-confidence. The competition involved in Initiative Group is always non-threatening. It is always team versus team, team versus the clock, team versus the problem or team versus its own past performance. It is never individual versus individual. If we do run into a situation where only two people are available for the group on a particular day, they either solve a problem together or are involved in something like a barrier activity (*Walkie Talkie Towers*), where both individuals are responsible for the success or failure.

The *physical challenge* involved in Initiative Group provides diversity from traditional, sit-down rehabilitation and from the rest of their therapeutic day. It also takes away from the school-like atmosphere, which can be very intimidating for some people.

Props, odd additions and *humor* help the clients to stand out from the crowd and to feel special. It adds fun to the group and provides relief from the constant serious focus of therapy. Many of the activities are presented within the context of a ridiculous story or setting. The serious part comes at the end, when we process how

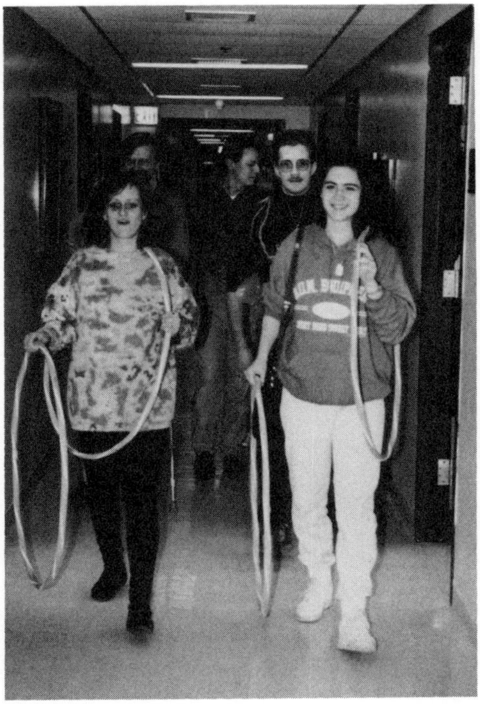

this crazy activity could have any bearing on real life. This fun attitude and the props also help to form more of a cohesive group.

Moderate structure is provided through closed-ended tasks and clearly stated goals and rules. It is also present in the three-stage Brief, Activity, Debrief format and performance prediction and evaluation that are a part of each and every group meeting.

The clients walk away with a feeling of *independence* in the sense that very little help is provided by the therapists during the actual performance of the activity. Instead, they are encouraged to rely on each other.

Everything related to the group is done or presented in a *positive way*. When negative feedback (constructive criticism) is given, it is provided on the heels of something positive that the person did. When the group fails, we discuss what changes they will make in order to come back and be successful next time. Or, we will talk about how terrific it is they could identify what was wrong with their performance. "No way" is answered with, "Absolutely," "No we can't" with, "Yes you can," and "I don't know how" is followed by, "...yet!" Sometimes we have been completely and pleasantly surprised by how addictive this attitude can be.

Conclusion

Chapter Two has focused on the important components of Initiative Group and specific adaptations that have made our group successful within our own facility. Consider how they relate to your setting and your population, then develop your own goals for group and admission criteria. Once this foundation is set, consult the six key elements just discussed when planning activities and setting the overall attitude of the group.

Chapter Three

Modifying Activities

We all deal with modification in our daily lives, some days more than others. Consider this day: You wake up late, but that's okay — you've already planned what you're going to wear. You go to the closet and find that the yellow shirt you wanted is in the laundry. So you decide to make a fashion statement and pull out a purple one instead. You head downstairs for your bowl of cereal only to find that someone left the milk out over night and now even the cat won't go near it. You grab a banana and head out the door.

The car practically steers itself along the usual route until you hear that the road you need is backed up with bumper to bumper traffic. No problem, you know an alternate route. Halfway to work you remember that you are out of dog food. You rummage around the front seat searching for a pen and paper. Finding neither, you grab a napkin and your favorite teal eyeliner and write yourself a note to buy the dog some food.

You make it through the rest of the day rather uneventfully except for a couple of comments about your new outfit. You make a mental note to go out on that fashion limb again. You arrive home only to be greeted by a hungry dog and you remember that you forgot to stop at the store. You grab the leftover spaghetti from the refrigerator and put it in his bowl. If he could purr he would — he never liked that canned stuff anyway!

Luckily, most days run more smoothly than this, but the need for a little modification generally creeps into each day. The same is true for Initiative Group.

Who Can Use Initiative Group

With a little modification, most of our activities can fit the goals of nearly all the therapeutic disciplines and can meet the needs of most challenged populations. Professionals from varied disciplines use the same activity, but for a different purpose and with a different emphasis. Also, the briefing and debriefing stages might be different.

For example, a counselor might use the group for clients who have difficulty expressing their feelings or forget how they feel when not actually involved in the activity. So their emphasis would be, "How did it feel to have to trust others? How did it feel to use your strategies with others watching? How did it feel to fail; to succeed?" And so on.

A neuropsychologist or a cognitive therapist will select the activities that have a greater problem solving element (or organization, sequencing planning, etc.).

A physical therapist will choose activities focusing on balance, coordination and endurance.

In some settings, vocational therapists might run the group and focus on teamwork and appropriate work behaviors.

Occupational therapists will choose those activities that have a greater need for fine motor skills, scanning and other visual perceptual skills.

Speech language pathologists would focus on group communication skills, including: social appropriateness, auditory comprehension and verbal expression.

Other disciplines that have expressed an interest in this approach include: education specialists, physical educators and therapeutic recreation specialists.

Who can Benefit from Initiative Group

This model can be applied to the following challenged populations:

- Traumatic Brain Injury
- Stroke
- Alzheimer's
- Multiple Sclerosis
- Muscular Dystrophy
- Spinal Cord Injury
- Amyotrophic Lateral Sclerosis
- Psychiatric

In addition, the model can be applied to people who are:

- Communicatively impaired
- Physically impaired
- Hearing impaired/deaf
- Visually impaired/blind
- Sensory impaired
- Neurologically impaired
- Orthopedically impaired
- Cognitively impaired
- Learning disabled
- Developmentally delayed
- Psychologically/socially impaired
- Mentally handicapped
- At risk for learning/language/physical/sensory difficulties
- Non-English speakers
- Low-English proficiency

Considerations

Modifying the activities to fit the population and adjusting them to further meet the needs of the individual group members is a fun and challenging part of the group for its leaders. Sometimes you will have the luxury of time and be able to anticipate the needs of your group and plan the necessary changes before the group begins. Other times, however, you will need to change things quickly, in the moment, as you see that the activity, or some aspect of it, is too easy or too hard for the group. In the twentieth anniversary issue of *Zip Lines* (Fall, 1991), Project Adventure's newsletter, Jim Grout, the Director of the PA Vermont office, reminds us that, "...the best adventure programming is only half planned." He continues, "The other half comes from the particular needs of those with whom we work. It is our ability to adapt our bag of tricks to a situation that is our expertise rather than to crank out a factory-honed adventure experience."

Analyze

Assuming that you already know the main emphasis of your group (communication, cognition, physical therapy, etc.), the first step in planning is to analyze the strengths, weaknesses and limitations of your individual group members. Remember to look at their physical, cognitive, psychological and communicative needs and abilities. If you need to, ask questions of other therapists, especially the physical therapist and counselor.

Once you have this information, choose an activity that will address your goal areas, yet has the potential to accommodate any client restrictions. When deciding whether an activity can be modified to meet your needs, first determine what aspect of the activity is too hard or too easy. Is it its physical, cognitive, psychological or communicative requirements? Then break it down further:

For **Physical Status** consider

- balance
- vestibular status
- visual perception
- fine motor control
- gross motor control
- ambulation status
- sensation
- safety awareness
- endurance

For **Cognitive Status** consider

- attention
- memory
- initiation
- safety awareness
- problem solving
- divergent thinking
- self-monitoring
- awareness of deficits
- impulsivity
- planning
- organization

For **Psychological Status** consider

- emotional ability to give feedback
- emotional ability to receive feedback
- ability to deal with failure
- stage in the adjustment process

For **Communication Status** consider

- expressive language
- receptive language
- reading
- writing
- pragmatic skills (how they interact with other people)

Group Versus Individual Changes

Once you have pinpointed the problem, decide whether the change should be instituted for an individual or for the group as a whole. The decision will be easy if the activity is too hard or easy for the *entire* group. You simply modify it for the group.

But if only one or two individuals will have difficulty with it or will solve it too quickly, the decision becomes more complex. You will need to decide whether to have the changes affect everyone or just those individuals. Your decision will depend on the individual the accommodation is for and the nature of the change. For instance, making overt special accommodations for someone who is temporarily in a wheelchair because of a broken leg can feel less threatening to him than to someone who is permanently in a wheelchair because of decreased motor control. For the person with the broken leg, you may decide to make the change just for him because he will be comfortable with the special treatment. However, if you need to work around the person who is permanently in a chair, you might decide to have everyone do the activity sitting down. In this way, you are not singling him out as different and you are also sending him the message that he can still be successful in his chair. Another reason to make a group change would be if the individual change or no change at all would put that person at an unfair disadvantage.

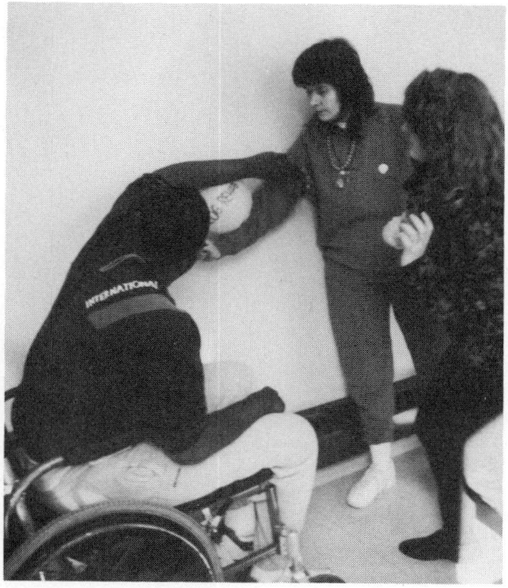

You'll find that very often you can work in an individual change without his even knowing it. As an example, you can set up a passing line with the person with one-sided weakness at the end of the line. In this way, his needing to use two hands never becomes an issue. Or, when handing out props, you can hand a large grip item to the person with decreased fine motor control. Whenever possible (which is most of the time), we are up-front about the special accommodations and why they are necessary. This approach normalizes the disability, sends the message that there is nothing wrong with it, and helps clients to understand what changes they will have to make in their lives.

Physical Modifications

There are many ways of adjusting activities to fit physical needs. Here are just a few.

Make the print larger
Wear blindfolds

To compensate for visual acuity deficits affecting reading, simply make the print larger. For activities like *Road Trip* and *Who's Driving That Car,* the "license plates" can all be written in standard sized print on a piece of paper; they can be written larger on individual index cards; or they can even be written very large on a blackboard. Vision can also be altered by having clients wear blindfolds.

CAUTION: Blindfolding is an excellent way of increasing the demands on visualization, communication, problem solving, balance and trust, but it eliminates clients' use of vision as a way of compensating for balance deficits. Many clients who have impaired motor and/or vestibular systems often rely heavily on their vision to maintain their balance. Under normal circumstances, you may not even be aware that someone's balance system is impaired because they compensate so well. Consult with the physical therapist before blindfolding a client. But just because someone does compensate well for balance with their vision does not mean that they cannot be blindfolded (unless the PT says no), you just have to be prepared to spot them according to their needs.

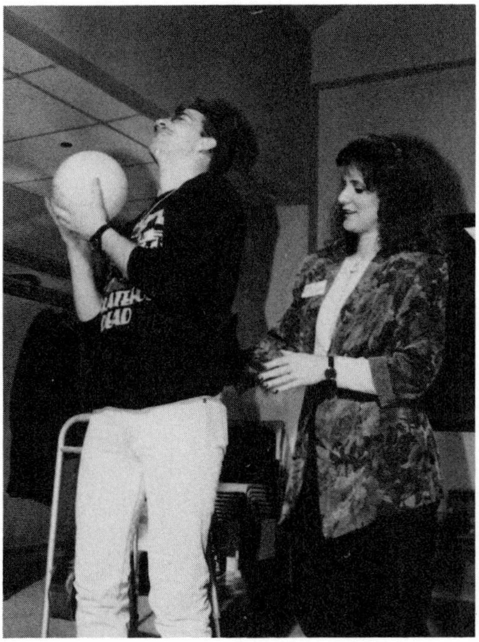

Keep eyes closed without blindfold
Keep eyes open and look at the floor

We use blindfolding a tremendous amount because it forces increased reliance on verbal communication, and we have many clients with balance problems who compensate with their vision. We just make sure that we know ahead of time who to be extra careful with and we always have enough spotters available. Occasionally, we have clients who are actually afraid of being blindfolded because of how they're going to feel. This may sound extreme to someone who has never experienced the feeling, since all they will be doing in some cases is standing still or taking a few small steps. But they may experience dizziness, nausea, double vision and headaches. Often, these symptoms can last for several hours. In those cases, we allow participants to keep their eyes closed without the blindfold. This way they have greater control and can open their eyes anytime they feel they are going to fall or feel nauseated. On one occasion, in fact, a young woman's balance was so poor without her vision that we allowed her to keep her eyes open and look at the floor. This modification worked very well, and she recognized these activities as adjuncts to her physical therapy sessions.

Use only one arm

Having the entire group use only one arm will also increase physical demands. It is a good rule to impose if you have someone who has one-sided weakness or paralysis and would be at a significant disadvantage without this rule. It gives others an understanding of this type of deficit as well. And, in most cases, it forces interaction with others. Have you ever tried to tie a tennis racket to a piece of wood with one hand by yourself? (See *Junkyard Swing*)

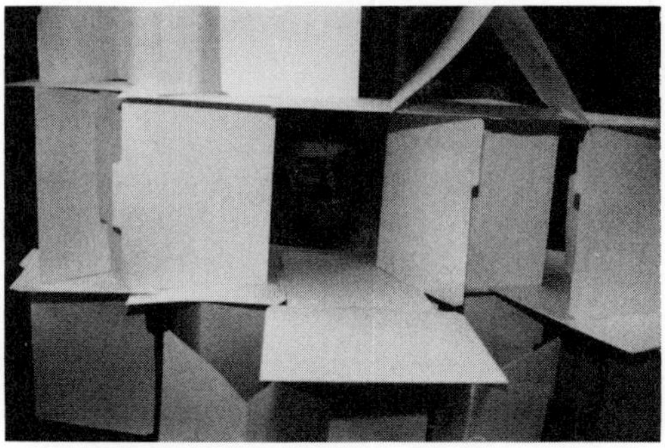

Use big or small props
Perform activities on uneven surfaces

Other ways of altering physical demands are to use big or small props as mentioned earlier (see *Walkie Talkie Towers*), and to perform activities on uneven surfaces (grass, hills, etc.). The size of props will shift the emphasis from fine motor (smaller props) to gross motor (larger). Heavier props can help to minimize the effects of ataxia (shaking), possibly allowing an ataxic person to participate in an otherwise unmanageable activity. As with blindfolds, varying the terrain can be dangerous for physically challenged people. Consult with the physical therapist for the go-ahead and for possible spotting and cueing techniques.

Sit or stand
Change positioning

Two other physical options available are sitting versus standing, and positioning. If your clients are in wheelchairs or cannot stand long enough to complete the activity, see if there is a way for the person or the group to do it sitting down. Or build in rest breaks. These breaks can be sneaked in or perhaps made overt in order to reinforce that the client will need to initiate them on his own when he is out in the community. Positioning can also be overt or covert as needed. The example of placing a hemiplegic at the end of a line given earlier was an example of positioning. Another example would be placing someone with a left-sided visual neglect on the right of all the action so that he would be forced to scan left.

The possibilities for physical modifications of the activities are endless, as they are in all of the other areas. Adjust as necessary and remember to pull in the occupational therapists and physical therapists when in doubt. If they are not available, err on the side of caution.

Cognitive Modifications

If you determine that the cognitive demands are what need to be modified, consider some of these ideas.

Cue clients to take notes

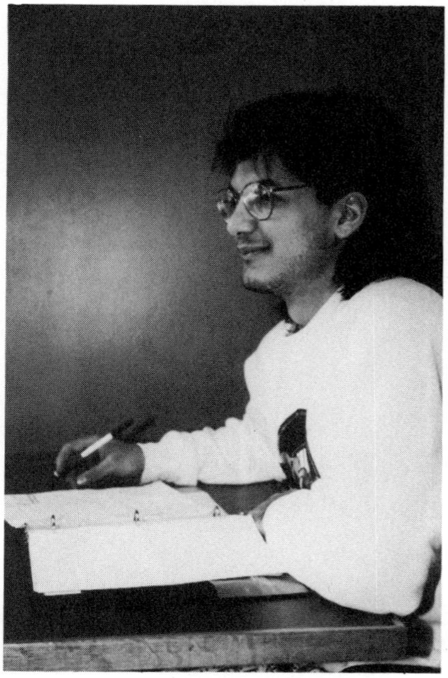

If memory is the area of difficulty, cue the clients to take notes. Of course you could — and we often do — not mention this and let the group fail by not taking notes and then have them discuss the problem during the debrief. Present the same activity, another version of it, or a similar one next time and see if they make the change and initiate note taking. If taking notes would be too difficult, you can give them written directions or rules. Sometimes we give the entire group only one set of directions to encourage communication. If someone suggests running out to make extra copies, we typically allow it since the idea represents Initiative, recognition of a potential difficulty, and good problem solving. Other times, *everyone* in the group gets a copy of the directions so that everyone is more clearly responsible for seeing that they are adhered to.

Allow clients to ask questions
Limit questions

Most of the time, we allow our group members to ask questions throughout the activity, since that's a strategy we want to reinforce. But if we want to stress planning ahead, anticipating problems and independent decision making, we limit questions to the first few minutes. If we choose this route, we usually let them know right up front (see procedures for *Pile-On*).

Alter the number of rules and props

There are some activities where more props make it easier (*Chain Reaction*), and some where less are easier (*Pile-On, Pack Your Bags*). The same idea goes for the number of rules. In some cases, rules help to provide structure, reduce ambiguity and sometimes help to point out the correct problem-solving path. In other cases, more rules mean more information to retain and more self-monitoring.

Use blindfolds

Using blindfolds, as discussed under *Physical Modifications* (see Caution), greatly increases the cognitive challenge, especially with respect to visualization and memory. For a lower level group, cueing clients to plan their strategy before they put the blindfolds on might mean the difference between success and failure (remember that failure is often a strong learning experience — don't be afraid to use it wisely). Making them plan after the blindfolds are on greatly increases the communicative demand as well.

Present the most challenging version first

For high level groups, you may present the most challenging version of an activity first. For instance, we have most groups solve *Blind Knots* (*Silver Bullets,* pgs. 117–118) with their eyes open first. Then they can use that experience to solve it while blindfolded. But if we felt we had a very high level group, we would have them attempt to solve it blindfolded and then back off to the easier version if we needed to.

Predict number of rule violations

To increase the group members' self-monitoring abilities, have them predict the number of rule violations they think they will commit. They can write their predictions down on their goal sheets or rule sheets. Building this process into all activities that have rules increases their awareness and reinforces the idea of self-monitoring more effectively.

Give the group responsibility for generating modifications

A fun way to challenge divergent thinking skills is to give the group responsibility for generating modifications. If there is time, they can try their idea out immediately, or you can make the brainstorming part of the debriefing process and plan a date to try the new game. If you have a very high level group, try *Gamemaster.*

Psychological Modifications

Assessing where to go with psychological changes is the most difficult determination — at least for us non-counselors. It is so important to get the best handle possible on where your clients are psychologically, including what stage in the adjustment process they are in. Be aware that if the deficits were acquired later in life (as opposed to being congenital), that their recovery may be complicated by psychological problems from before their injury or illness. This pre-morbid functioning will likely greatly influence their post-injury coping style.

Adjust the level of emotional exposure
Cue, structure and time feedback
Emphasize group performance

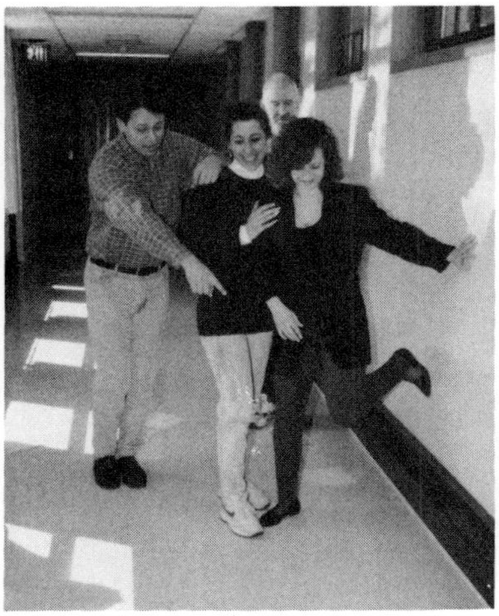

Consulting with a client's counselor will help you to tune into the individual's needs and better grasp how much challenge and reality (or direct feedback) should be incorporated into the activity or debrief. The PA concept lends itself to situations that promote successful experiences within an environment of alternating levels of emotional safety. You, as the group facilitator, may adjust the level of emotional exposure to suit your clients through cues, structure and timing of feedback. For example, generous cueing and structure may be appropriate to build a successful experience for a member with low confidence and high fear of failure. Likewise, emphasis on group performance as opposed to individual skills eases pressure on those self-doubters and increases their willingness to risk and share their skills and ideas. This safety net of group goals buffers the hurt of failure as it is now perceived as shared failure, while sending the message that no one is expected to be perfect.

Use the Adventure Wave
Focus on positive actions
Address failure issues
Encourage feedback from peers
Follow up in an individual session
Lessen the focus on winners and losers

Debriefing is an important follow-up for all experiences — whether they be perceived failures or successes. Review the group's achievements using the Adventure Wave concept, which focuses on learning from past experiences to improve future performance. There is always another opportunity to succeed. We will take what we learned today, apply it to tomorrow and will succeed eventually. Style your debrief to focus either on more positive actions or to more confrontively address failure issues depending on the level of feedback your client is ready to manage. Often, group feedback from peers rather than therapists can be less confrontive, while at other times, one may be more comfortable with following up in an individual session with the group's leader. (Keep in mind that some clients don't know how to give feedback in a diplomatic fashion or are unaware of how they are perceived. Be prepared to jump in and soften the blow if you use this approach.) You can lessen the focus on winners and losers by setting up an activity as a competition but then eliminating score keeping (as in *Blind Spear Fishing* and *Wetdown*). Allow them to just get caught up in the experience and have fun.

As a rule of thumb, if you are not sure of the impact an Initiative will have on the group or on an individual, don't do it. Wait until they are ready or check with the counselor to get more input. There are plenty of other Initiatives to choose from. Psychological damage can take a long time to reverse. It's not worth the risk.

Communicative Modifications

We are finally at the area where we're experts. Well, at least, the area where we like to think we're experts!

Institute communication rules

In order to make the group members more aware of others and to increase communication, we have two general rules that are part of every activity:

1. Individual plans must be communicated to the group prior to taking action (speak before you act);
2. Each group member must be actively aware of and involved in the plan at all times.

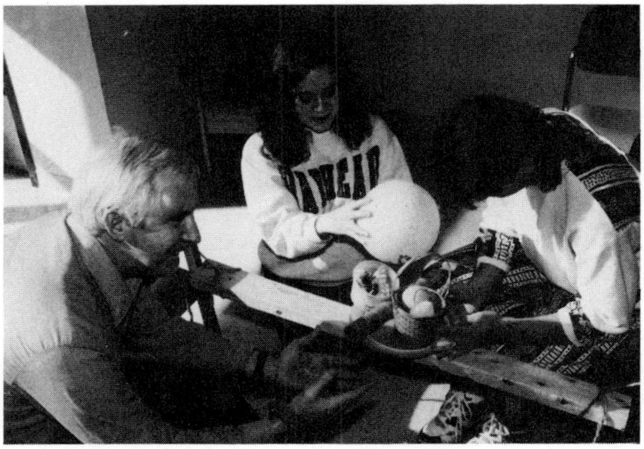

Rule number one can become a naturally learned behavior with repetitive cues. Rule number two, however, presents more of a challenge to our head injured groups, who typically have significantly decreased auditory comprehension and initiation. Noncompliance with this rule results in lost members quietly interest in the task. Use this moment to be the first to put their thoughts into words. With your best puzzled expression ask, "Why in the heck would we make you wear blindfolds? When in the 'real world' would you ever be in a situation like this?" Exaggerate your intonation when you ask this question like even you recognize that its the stupidest thing you could ever ask them to do. An answer, by the way, is the telephone. It's a situation where you are essentially blindfolded, needing to rely solely on verbal communication. We have never had anyone ever continue to question the blindfolds after this discussion.

Use barrier activities
Encourage note taking

Barrier activities increase demands in a way similar to blindfolds. In barrier games, two teams work together to each construct an identical end product. The barrier placed between the teams blocks the use of vision and gestures, thereby placing emphasis solely on clear, direct verbal communication (*Walkie Talkie Towers*). In these activities, the responsibility for an accurate replica lies with both sides, not just the direction givers. The receivers are also responsible for asking as many clarifying questions as needed. Other activities may encourage note taking as a strategy to compensate for memory deficits or practice writing skills. Your group's goals will dictate where the emphasis will be.

Add rules calling for cooperative efforts

Another way of increasing communicative demands is to increase the complexity of the task with additional rules that call for cooperative efforts and active problem solving among group members. In *Move It or Lose It* they can hand items to other people, but they cannot pick up the prop that they are ultimately going to carry. This rule led to a big dilemma for one group that could not figure out how they were going to get props to the final person without dropping anything they were already carrying. They never did figure it out.

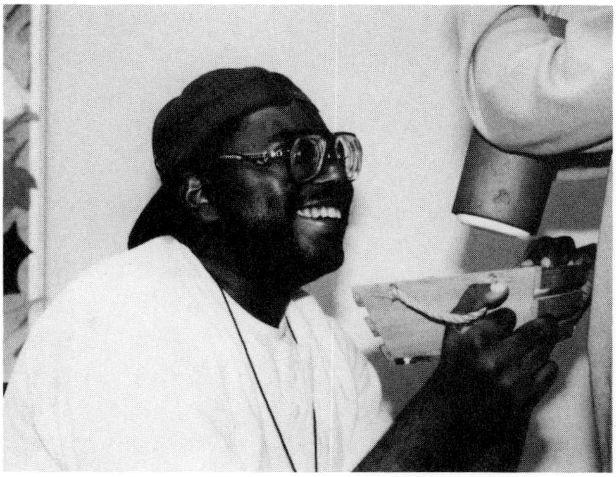

Require explanation of decisions and performance

We've found that an effective summary flows from asking clients to verbally explain and defend their decisions and performance. This challenge to defend their solutions makes sure that:

1. they can remember their reasons
2. they weighed their options and formulated a rational decision.

This method works well for activities like *Fillet of Sole* and *Who's Driving That Car*? A subtle variation of this idea is to have them retell the steps in order of what they did and why with games like *Pile-on, Pack Your Bags* and *Mystery Box Rescue*. This technique lends itself as an excellent lead-in to the debriefing process.

Modifications,Variations, and Versions

At the end of several of the activities, there is a section labeled *Modifications*. There you will find some ways we have adapted that particular activity to match our members' needs. You may find them helpful, too. Several of the activities have a section or sections labeled *Variations*. These are different from the modifications because their intention is not to compensate for deficits. They are simply different ways of doing the activity. These variations are often good to use on another day to assess the transfer of skills learned from the first activity to the variation.

You will also find that in some cases there will be more than one version of an activity. This version is written up separately as a stand alone activity because it was different enough from the original that it could be performed instead of the original. Typically, we utilize these second versions when the group has finished the first one too quickly. All the props and main setups are generally the same, so all you have to do is give the new instructions. A good example of this is *Pile-On* and *Pile-On Competition*.

Safety

We have mentioned safety several times throughout this chapter, especially as it relates to the physical and emotional realms. To someone trained in working with non-disabled people on Project Adventure's high ropes courses or Outward Bound's wilderness survival expeditions, a discussion about safety involving Initiative Group's activities might seem unnecessary, given their comparatively low intensity. But safety truly is an issue. Consider that standing still or walking even a few steps may be unsafe activities for some people. We've worked with many people who have been terrified to take a couple of steps even with someone holding onto them because it makes them feel out of control and unsafe. So for them *challenge* and *risk* take on whole new meanings than they do for the rest of us. We need to acknowledge and respect these feelings when working with differently-abled populations.

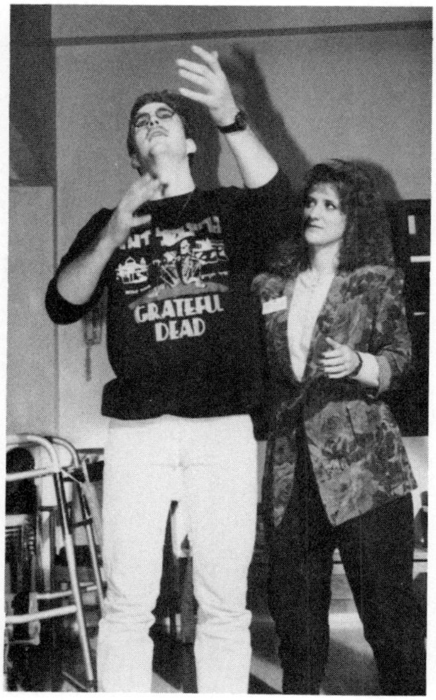

Admittedly, too, our willingness as leaders to place some of these people in risky situations is lessened given what some of them have recently been through. They may have multiple healing or recently healed fractures, cuts, bruises and internal injuries. Reinjury could set them back months in their rehabilitation. Many of the people we work with have just come from being in the hospital for weeks or months. The last thing that we want is for them to end up back there. Also, our clients with physical deficits or injuries tend to be very focused on their bodies, as is only natural at that stage in their recovery. So this means that even minor scratches, aches and pains tend to be overly focused on. For some, even a minor mishap might result in their refusal to continue to participate in the group. So, we choose our challenges very carefully with safety as our first concern and abide by the philosophy of Challenge By Choice. This doesn't mean that we don't challenge them, it just means that we need to find out what is challenging to them *now*, soon after a traumatic and perhaps life-threatening event. Our goal is to first increase their self-esteem and knowledge about what they are capable of doing. Then we can increase the level of challenge and risk as they are ready for it.

You need to determine what kinds of risks the people you work with can handle given how and when they became disabled. A group of developmentally disabled people may be open to more risk (or may not!). Listen to your group. Weigh your risks carefully.

Below is a list of some safety considerations common to many rehabilitation populations.

1. As mentioned before, keep in mind that blindfolding may exacerbate balance, dizziness and nausea symptoms. Always check in with the physical therapist and the client to get an idea of what to expect.
2. Clearly know any and all medical histories, physical limitations and potential problems for all clients in the group. This would include:
   - Comfortable and safe range of motion
   - Allergies — including bee stings if you will be working outdoors
   - Weight bearing status
   - Status with transfers (contact guard, close supervision, independent, etc.)
   - Ambulation status on various terrain — independent inside on hard floors may not mean independent outside on grass
   - Cardiac or respiratory precautions
   - History of seizures, etc.
   - Medication schedule

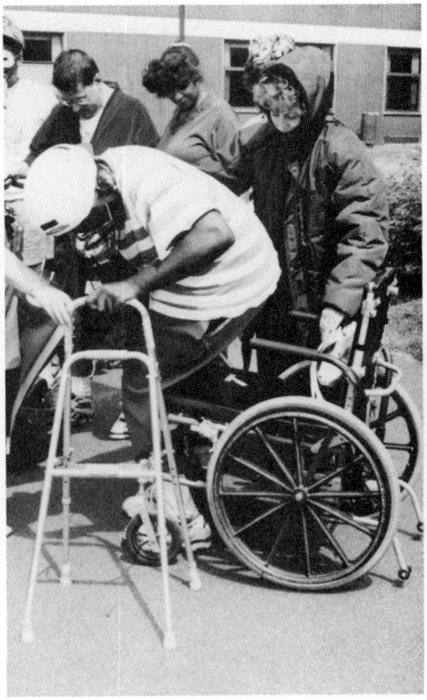

3. Know how to transfer someone from the floor to standing or to a chair.
4. Know how to guard (spot) someone standing or ambulating. Here is a general grading system that we use. From what we hear, this terminology is pretty standard in physical therapy circles. Thanks to Barbara Surhoff, B.S., P.T. for making it clear to us. Unless you are a P.T., you aren't likely to be responsible for determining a grading for someone, but knowing the P.T.'s terminology will help facilitate communication. When in doubt, ask them to demonstrate what they mean. Actually being trained with the particular client may make you and him more confident when the need presents itself in the group.

Hands-On Assistance

Dependent: Client performs 0% of the activity. He will need the maximum amount of support.

Maximum assist: Client performs 25% of the activity. You will need to provide direct hands-on assistance most of the time in order for the client to perform the activity safely.

Moderate assist: Client performs 50% of the activity. Again, a hands-on approach is used to maximize safety.

Minimum assist: Client performs 75% of the activity while the therapist maintains hands-on contact.

Contact Guard
Assistance in maintaining balance is infrequently provided by the therapist, however, hands-on contact is maintained to maximize safety.

Supervision
The therapist may need to provide verbal cues, but no-hands on assistance is required.

Independent
No intervention is needed for safe performance.

5. Cue to lock wheelchair brakes when appropriate
6. Know that some body positions or movements may increase symptoms of vertigo or nausea
7. Know that heat may increase the likelihood of seizures, fainting, etc.
8. Know your facility's medical emergency protocol but hope that you will never need it!

This list is far from complete. Take some time to consider safety with each new activity and each new set of individuals before and during the activity. Reflect back afterwards and decide whether there was anything you would change in the future. There is a very fine line between challenge and unacceptable risk. When that line becomes unclear, choose safety first.

Conclusion

If, after reading an activity, your first reaction is, "I can't do that with my group," or "Not while so-and-so is in the group," look again. Most likely there is a way of modifying it to compensate for varying deficits and needs. Use the ideas from this chapter to help guide your thinking, and always put safety first.

For further information regarding safety and current standards, see Project Adventure's *Ropes Course Safety Manual.*

Chapter Four

Practical Considerations

Now for a few words on logistics. Some of these things we considered initially, before beginning the group, but most of them we stumbled across as the need arose. For example, we didn't think about putting all of the rule sheets and attendance lists we were accumulating into a three-ring binder until the fourth time they all fell out of our folder as we were walking to group. Four times were enough. We learned. The binder really has made life easier.

Before beginning your group, read this chapter carefully and consider how these issues will relate to your facility, group, clients and co-leaders. It may take some time to establish your own routine and to become comfortable. But don't worry, it will come.

Spread the Word

Inform others — both the staff and administration — about the new group. Let them know what to expect to see. They may see people walking down the hallways with strange things in their hands or on their heads. They may see clients searching in odd places like the change slot of the pay phone. They may see you walking around armed with a bag of water balloons and some lunch trays. They may even see people having fun! (Gasp!)

You can inform staff during an inservice or a staff meeting. Remember that this is a nontraditional approach in rehabilitation and that there might be some attitudes to overcome. In our facility everybody pretty much said, "Sounds great," and we were on our way! Take this opportunity to teach them about Project Adventure and experiential learning theory so they know there is a therapeutic purpose to all they'll see. You might even lead them through a few activities, including briefing and debriefing.

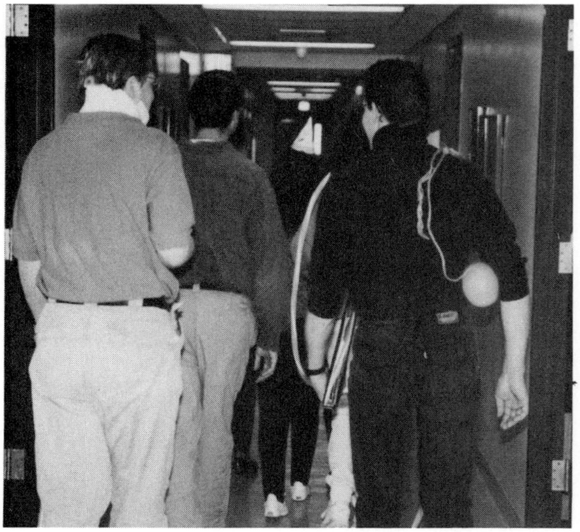

Get the Lay of the Land

Know where you can and cannot do things and at what times. Look both inside and outside. You are looking for things like big rooms, blank walls, long hallways, playgrounds and basketball courts. Figure out when they are free. In the case of hallways, learn the traffic patterns. Using the hallway near the cafeteria during peak snack time may not be ideal.

Be Comfortable

Getting completely comfortable with the group and all of its various aspects takes time. However, there are some things you can do to maximize your comfort level on that very first day.

Understand the theory and concepts behind experiential learning and PA. Know these well so that when you need to present or do something in a goofy way, you will clearly know the goal of it and could explain it if challenged. Be comfortable in the knowledge that what you are doing is therapeutic, albeit a bit nontraditional.

Be comfortable with your co-leader. It's important to be comfortable with your co-leader in any type of group situation, but it is especially important with this type of content. Your relationship is going to grow and gel over time, but you can help push it in the right direction from the beginning. Make sure you have definite times to get together and talk about the group. Agree, before there are any problems to discuss, to give and receive feedback openly between each other. Make sure that you both have the same ideas about where the group is, where you want it to go, and what the overall goals are.

Be comfortable doing goofy things and presenting them in a goofy way. If you are not comfortable, the clients won't be. Understanding *why* you are doing something can go a long way toward making you more at ease. Recognize that all your clients will not always feel comfortable doing things that are a little out of the ordinary. Prepare them by explaining right up front that they will be participating in a session that is different from others. Doing so right off will help them to relax and "go with it." Also, make both the group goals and the individual goals very clear, and refer to them frequently so that the clients understand that there is a purpose behind these new activities. We do believe in F.U.N.N. (functional understanding not necessary), but have found that in rehabilitation, our *clients* do not always believe the same way. Besides, we have also seen that the greater the understanding the clients have about why they are doing something, the greater the changes they can make.

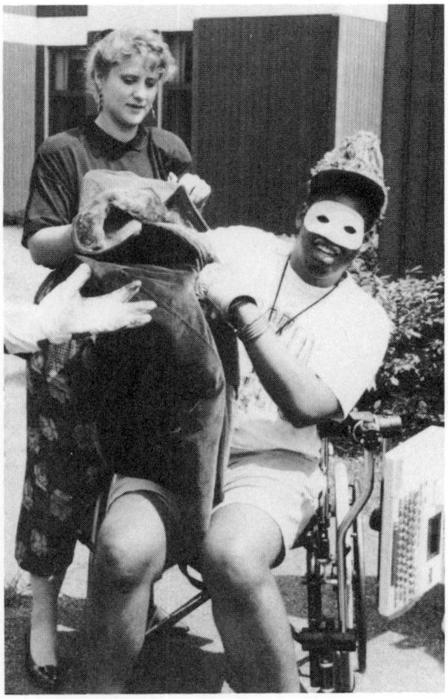

In addition to seeing increased clinical change, it is hoped that an understanding of what is happening and why will head off direct challenges. But be prepared for them. Working with cognitively impaired clients, we tend to get challenged from time to time because they cannot always abstract and see the purpose in what we ask them to do. Most of the time we can defuse these challenges by turning it right back to them: "That's a good question; why *are* we doing this?" It is much better if support for the activity can come from that client or from his peers rather than from the leaders. On other occasions, when the clients felt the activity was too easy (even when we didn't always agree), we challenged them to modify it to make it more difficult. One day we even ended an activity mid-stream and moved on to something completely different, because we agreed with them that we had made a wrong decision in choosing the activity. The ultimate goal is to be in tune with your group and not be put in this position in the first place. But if you do make a mistake, don't try to plod through and make it work; it won't. And you will end up losing more than you will have gained. This flexibility sends a couple of strong messages. It lets the clients know that they do have some control in this process, and it tells them that we respect their ideas.

If all else fails and we cannot help an individual group member to understand an activity when everyone else does, we remind them that everything in group is Challenge by Choice, and they are welcome to sit this one out and just watch. Given this choice, most have opted to continue — without further resistance.

Lastly, be comfortable within your facility with non-group colleagues. By educating them beforehand and knowing how best to use your physical layout, you shouldn't get too many odd looks.

Props

One day it occurred to us that many of our activities involved props. Some of them even have substantial lists of added items. We thought this odd, so we sat down to develop a bunch of non-prop tasks. After sitting awhile and thinking without too much to show for ourselves, we decided to do two things. One was to look at what purpose our props were serving, and two was to analyze why we weren't using more of PA's non-prop or low-prop activities.

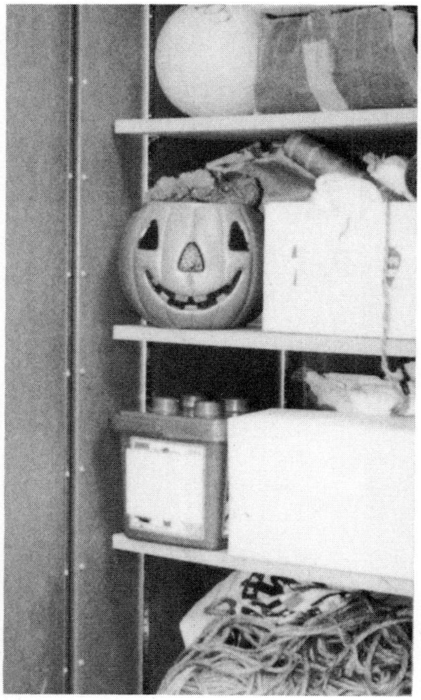

What we learned was that the props allowed us to maintain a cognitive challenge while limiting the physical demands. Props also provided us with a way of doing some of PA's activities that would otherwise be too difficult. Consider PA's *The Wall* (*Cowstails and Cobras II*, pgs. 113–115). We loved the idea, but there is no way we can have our clients helping each other over a 12-foot wall (too many monetary and physical constraints). However, we can have them get objects up and over a piece of rope (see *Balloom*). *Balloom*, with its several props, affords us a way of doing a great PA activity.

So what should you do? Grab a box or a cabinet somewhere and begin gathering crazy stuff everywhere you go — rubber chickens, plastic dinosaurs, slinkies, trolls. Don't worry, you don't need to have a purpose for it now, one will come to you later. Many of our activities involve props, but they rarely have to be specific items. Use whatever you have and relax! Be flexible. Before we had a stockpile of our own, we used to run around our office borrowing stupid things from people's desks (volleyball trophy, Mardi Gras beads, rulers, yo-yos, whistles). You'd be surprised how much we were able to find!

Your box should have in it just a few basic items that you will see used over and over:

- rope — various lengths
- blindfolds
- hoola hoop
- balloons
- balls
- basket or bucket — something with a handle that you can put things in. We use a plastic trick-or-treat pumpkin!
- slime (hand cream) — what good box o' stuff would be complete without it?

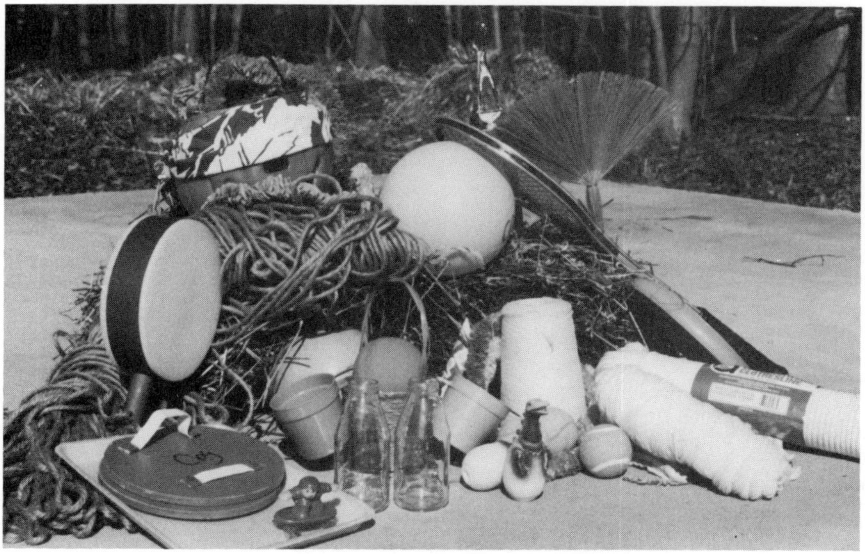

A general rule of thumb when selecting props: the funnier or more ridiculous the better.

There are some activities that do require specific props that you may not want to keep in the box all the time, like your spouse's clothing for *Dressing Relay Race*. Since to be really effective Initiative Group requires planning ahead, you should always know what you need long enough before the next group so that you will be ready. Plan far enough ahead so that you can get ready, but not so far that you become out of touch with where the group is at. Reassess your plan sometime before the group begins and consider any unscheduled absences or last minute admissions. Once you have done a certain activity one time, you will know what works and can quickly gather the necessary props again without too much additional thought.

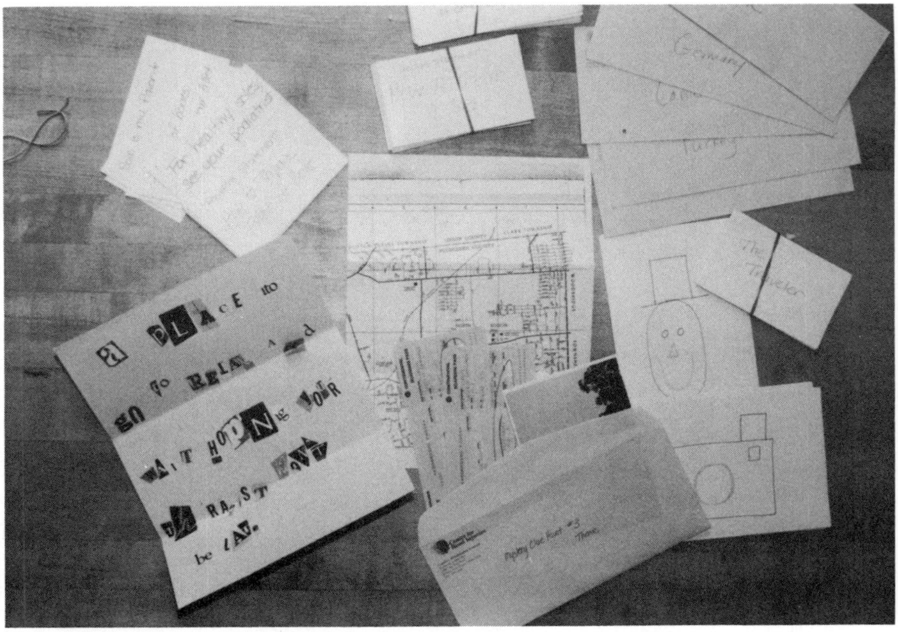

Other activities require specific cards like, *Drawing Relay Race* and *Fillet of Sole*. You should only need to make them once. Just make sure you write on index cards or cover them with contact paper so they are somewhat durable. Whenever practical, we try to present things in such a way that all you need to do is photocopy a page, like rules, and you are ready to go. If your rules are different from ours, write them out neatly or type them and always keep a few copies on hand in your notebook. Which brings up the idea of...

Organization

In a word or three — GET A NOTEBOOK! Since you are in a rehabilitation setting, your group is likely to be ongoing, with members coming and going as clinically appropriate and not necessarily at the same time, so you'll need a way of keeping track of them. Keep an attendance sheet that has their names across the top and a chronological list of activities down the side. Check off who participated in which activity. Then, when you are planning upcoming groups, you can easily scan the book and know which activities have been done by which people.

Make a section for activities. Keep the rule sheets that you have used, with multiple copies if you like. You can also keep the cards and other materials in it that aren't appropriate for the prop box.

It helps to have another section for goal sheets. Theoretically, our clients are responsible for making additional copies of their sheets so they never run out. Unfortunately, it doesn't always work out that way. You can use this section to quickly check out a client's goals or use the original to run off extra copies if needed.

Add other sections to the book as needed. Others might be medical information and emergency protocols.

Do it! You'll thank yourself later.

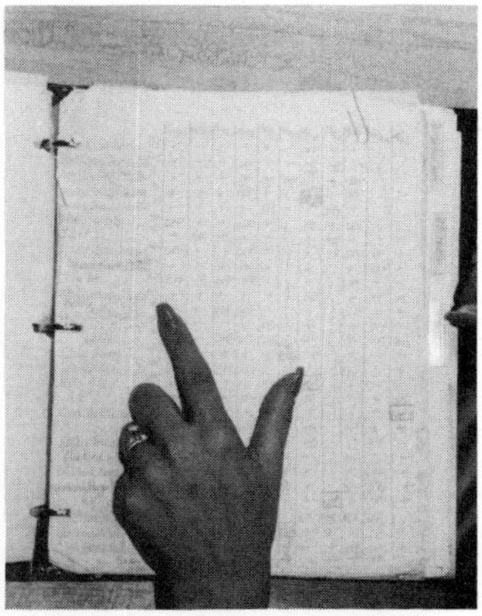

Fall-Back Positions

We recommend that you have a handful of quick, no-prop activities ready to go at all times. We use them when an activity takes less time than we planned and we are all out of different variations to try. Or, when an activity is just too frustrating and the group needs a quick, fun pick-me-up. Some that we find outstanding for this purpose are *Zen Clap*, *This Is My Nose*, and *Me Switch* (*More New Games*, 1981). With these activities, we focus on memory, learning and speed of processing. If you were planning on being outside, you may want to have an alternate on hand in case of inclement weather. Depending on your space constraints, many of the outdoor-type activities can be done indoors as well.

Conclusion

This chapter contains many of the things that have made our lives — at least with respect to Initiative Group — infinitely easier. Essentially, they can be summarized in four words: communication, understanding, organization and planning. We hope these work for you as well.

Section Two

Now, on to the fun! And we do mean fun! Don't forget to make fun an integral part of your sessions. Encouraging fun lightens the mood and reduces stress. We realize that this intentional inclusion of fun may not be a normal part of your therapy day. That's okay. Just go with it. Soon it will feel natural.

In this section you will find Initiatives uniquely designed for special populations. Become familiar with them and select the ones that are appropriate for meeting the goals you want to achieve. When presenting them, remember to keep the Adventure alive.

ALIEN INVASION

You need to do a little bit of running around for *Alien Invasion* before the group gathers. What you need to do ahead of time should become clear as you read on. If not, read this again. If it still doesn't make sense, then by all means, make something up!

Procedure

Before your group arrives in your usual meeting place, leave a ransom note on the table, like the one below, from an alien. It tells the group that one of their favorite therapists has been taken on an adventure and will be brought back, but the group must pick her up. You can use a more traditional kidnapping scenario if you like.

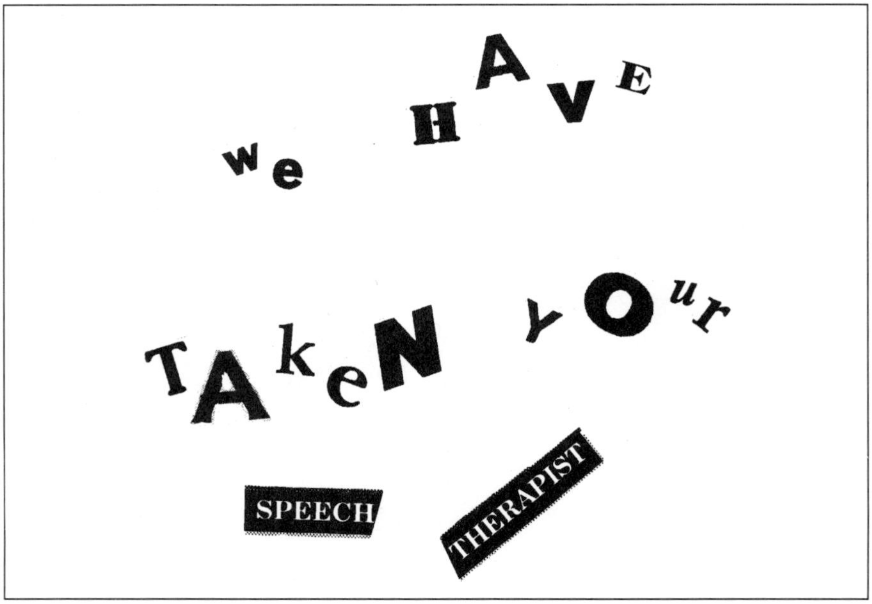

In order for the group to locate her, they must pull together to solve the clues that she has left behind. We invariably spend the first few minutes with the group deciding whether they really want to find the missing therapist or not!

Along with the ransom note, read to them a data sheet (or police report) put together from information from witnesses. This sheet should definitely include information about where the group should begin looking and what the therapist was wearing, but it should also have other irrelevant information (see example). You can hand the data sheet to them when you are done reading it so they can refer back to it, or have them rely on their own notes.

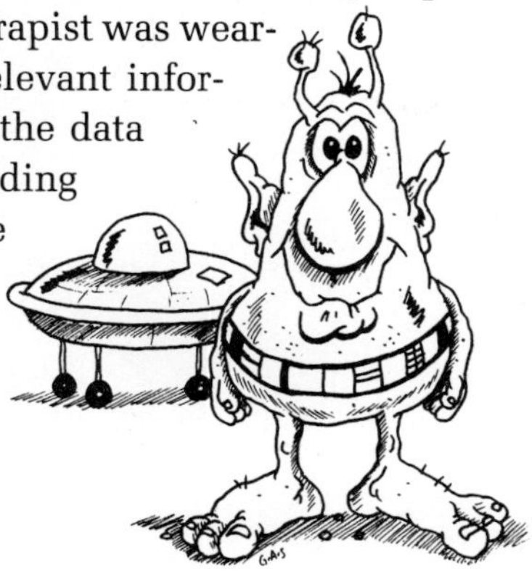

Police Report Data Sheet

Date:

Name of Missing Person:

Last Seen:

Comments: According to a co-worker, was wearing a red sweater, black slacks and white sneakers. An eyewitness reported that he saw her talking with alien-like creatures. They had oddly shaped heads, bulging eyes, bulbous noses and funny looking mouths. These beings stood about three-feet tall. The witness was quoted as saying, "The three of them were gone in a flash. One minute they were there and the next minute they were gone."

Two reliable witnesses reported that the therapist was last seen in the Great Room. She was wearing a red sweater and blue pants. She appeared to be relaxed. The witnesses left the room before the therapist and have not seen her again since that time.

When the group asks what they should do, shrug your shoulders and tell them that you don't know. You just know that it's really important for them to find her. Eventually they will look back to their clues and decide to head, in our case, to the Great Room. (In case you were wondering, the Great Room got its name because it is very big.) On a table in the Great Room, we leave an Initiative Group folder. You can be sure it's an IG folder because it has INITIATIVE GROUP written across it in big, bold letters. Inside the folder is an incomplete note from the therapist explaining that she will try to leave clues if she can. She writes that she overheard some information, but does not know what it means. She hopes that the information helps. We leave the letter of a wing in the building or a telephone extension. Of course, they are not told what this information represents — that is left for them to figure out.

In that next location, we leave red yarn in a trail to the next clue. Why red yarn? It's from the red sweater, of course. If you are wondering which red sweater, you read too fast. Go back and reread! The group follows the red trail and finally comes upon a note left by the aliens. It explains that the therapist is in a nearby room and tells what they must do to get her out. They must figure out a combination to unlock the door. The combination is in the form of a Magic Triangle. Along with the note are six circles with the numbers one through six on them. A triangle must be formed so that each side adds up to the same number.

After they solve the Magic Triangle they can open the door and find their therapist. But wait! What's this? She's blindfolded and behind a maze of tables and chairs. She must be verbally guided past them without touching anything before the blindfold can be removed.

If time is running short, the last part(s) can be left out (the combination or obstacle course). Save enough time to debrief.

As with other activities, you can make *Alien Invasion's* clues once and then use them over and over. We have found that it helps to label them with where they should be placed since you may not do this activity again for awhile. What took the most time during the preparation for us was deciding who got to sit in a treatment room for forty minutes getting caught up on paperwork. Let's be realistic...Initiative Group is fun, but a free session is a free session!

Skill Areas

The skills that *Alien Invasion* targets are going to depend, in part, on your choice of clues. You could substitute your own and make them all physically, verbally or visually based. In general, though, *Alien Invasion* will address problem solving, deductive reasoning, and attention to detail and communication. The activities that involve being up and moving around hallways also address impulsivity very well. This happens when the clients are encouraged to stay together and work as a group and not run off to pursue their own ideas.

Items Needed:

ransom note
folder
red or any color yarn
blindfold
data sheet
6 paper circles
note from therapist

Group Size: **2 or more**

Format: **Group**

ALL TIED UP

All Tied Up is a fun, low-prop activity which places the emphasis on visual problem solving and communication.

Procedure

For this game you will need one rope for every two people. If you have an odd number, have one of the leaders join in. Everyone stands in a circle. Give one end (and only one end at this point) of each rope to a different person. So, if you have eight people, you should have four ropes and four people holding onto one end of different ropes. The leaders take the four remaining ends and weave them in and out of each other into a tangled mess. Then they hand those four ends to the people without ropes. Now you should have eight people standing in a circle, probably looking a bit confused, holding the ends of ropes which lead into a muddled knot in the middle and then back out to who knows who.

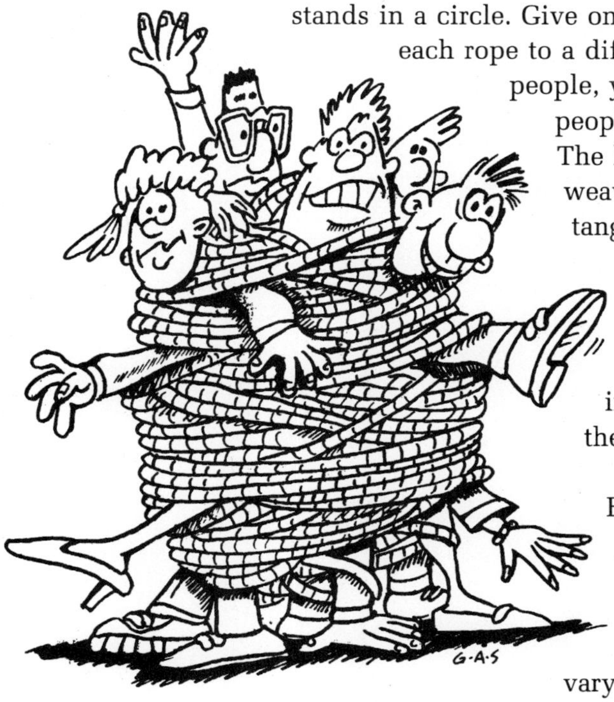

The group must untie the knot. But...there's a catch! Each person must stay with their end of the rope at all times. This means they will be climbing over, through and under the tangle. What's nice about *All Tied Up* is that you can vary the degree of difficulty of the knots for different level groups. People in wheelchairs should not have any difficulty participating. They can simply roll over the ropes rather than step over them.

The group may just need to make sure the opening is a little wider.

All Tied Up is good for problem solving, divergent thinking and frustration. Remember to encourage the group to communicate with each other.

SAFETY NOTE: People with significant balance problems may have difficulty with *All Tied Up.* This activity can serve as a good challenge for these clients, but you need to be prepared. You may decide not to have the leaders participate so they can serve as spotters. With some clients, it works to discuss potential difficulties and solutions after the instructions are given. In this way, you can get a lot of insight into their judgment and possible community safety. See if they can generate ideas like:

"I'll need to move slowly when I step over the rope."
"The rope will need to be flat on the ground."
"I'll need someone's hands on my hips."
"I'll need to hold onto someone's shoulder."
"I'll need to have one hand on my cane."

Variations

We generally just vary *All Tied Up* by increasing the complexity of the knot and have the group solve it a couple of times. You could, though, have them perform their feat blindfolded or without speaking. In either case, each person must communicate to the group what he is going to do before making a move.

Items Needed: **4 two-foot rope lengths**

Group Size: **4 or more**

Format: **Group**

BALLOOM

Balloom (not a spelling error!) is fun outdoors or in a big room like a gym. It brings a lot of skills together, including: eye/hand coordination, cooperation, attention and communication. It may not be appropriate for someone who has upper extremity (arm) ataxia (shaking), which cannot be controlled by an external stabilizer (wrist weight). Also think about where you set it up — on grass versus something like concrete — because it may affect the level of supervision a client requires when walking.

Procedure

Balloom uses two volleyball net poles without the net. Instead of the net, tie several ropes across from one pole to the other. When you are done it should look like a wide ladder. The top and bottom "rungs" can be as high and low as fits your group. If you are working with a group in wheelchairs, you would probably put the highest one at a comfortable stretch from chair height. They will be holding a paddle, so figure that in your height guesstimates. If your group is made up of people sitting *and* standing, you'll want to include some high and low rungs so everyone can be involved but also challenged.

Split the group in two and place the teams on opposite sides of the "ladder." Any type of ball will work, but we recommend the cheap, plastic kickball kind. Each person is given a paddle (racquet, bat, piece of wood, etc.). Using the paddles only, they must pass (not hit) a ball back and forth between the rungs, starting from the bottom, going to the top and coming back down. Each person must take a turn. If the ball drops and touches the ground, the group must start over at the bottom of the ladder. Optional rule: If the ball falls and is caught, they may begin at the level at which it was caught.

Modifications

You can make it a little different by sliding the knots up or down along the pole and making the ropes slanted. Then the group has to decide the best route. You can decide whether the ball is allowed to touch the rope or not or let the group set their own standard.

If your group becomes really good, you can challenge them by seeing how fast they can pass the ball up and down or how many balls they can have going at once. How about using water balloons on a hot summer day? You can also make *Balloom* more difficult by making the passing tool longer and thinner and by making the balls smaller. If your group has a lot of difficulty, let them use a partially deflated beach ball or a balloon.

So why the name *Balloom*? Well, someone noticed that it looked like a ball loom as the ball is passed back and forth between the ropes...get it?

Items Needed: **volleyball net poles**
rope
balls
paddles

Group Size: **2 or more**

Format: **Group**

BEND, BUMP AND ROLL

Bend, Bump and Roll places a big demand on divergent thinking, word finding and speed of processing skills. Despite the name, *Bend, Bump and Roll* does not require a lot of physical movement.

Procedure

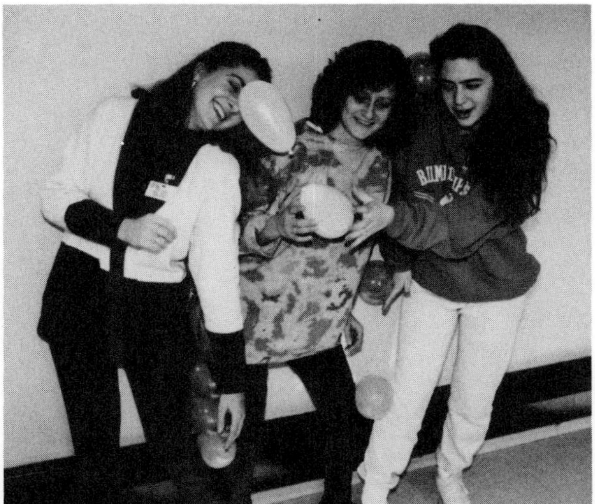

The group should be divided in half. The teams will need to sit or stand close together.

The game begins with a leader calling out one of the categories listed below. Some are fairly concrete and others are a little more abstract. At this point, anyone can shout out something that belongs in that category. The first one to shout out an acceptable word earns a point for their team. Then the other team has an opportunity to add one to the list. The teams alternate giving answers. The members of each team should go in a predetermined order so that everyone has their skills challenged. After attempting to think of an answer without success, others may give clues to their teammate, but may not give them the actual word. Set an appropriate time limit for a response. Thirty seconds works well for us. If the one team cannot generate a response in that time, the other team goes. Set a time limit for each category. Start with four minutes for the first few categories and then begin shortening them, finally ending up with one minute rounds. Whoever generates the most words in that round wins it. Have one of the leaders keep track of the number of words said by each team. If a word is repeated, they lose that turn and the other team goes. A longer time limit will challenge word finding and divergent thinking. Shorter rounds will emphasize speed of processing.

Each time a team wins a category, they are given a balloon. The team must hold the balloons between their bodies, not in their hands. For example, they can hold them shoulder to shoulder, leg to leg, etc. If a balloon falls, the other team has a chance to win it by naming another member of the most recent category (unless you happen to know what category the fallen balloon represents).

Water balloons would make this very interesting...

If competition of this sort wouldn't work well for your group, simply modify! For example, you might have the person switch teams each time he cannot generate an item. Of course, that leaves the problem of all the balloons he's holding between himself and his partners. He'd need to transfer them (no hands) to the partners before switching. In this way, the teams are constantly changing so there is no real winning or losing team. If it's likely that the same person or persons would be the only one(s) switching, then have a set position move; i.e., the person toward the front.

Categories

colors
fruits
vegetables
girls' names
boys' names
animals
cars
television shows
famous people
magazines
fabrics
fast food restaurants
subjects studied in school
occupations
things that are flexible
things that are frozen
things that you read
things that bounce

things that grow
things that are round
things that are heavy
things that make noise
things that you put in a box
things that have a strong odor
things that fly
things that teenagers say
things that descend
things in the refrigerator
things found in a junk drawer
reasons to celebrate
summer sports
types of food
types of dessert
words that describe things made of glass
reasons to take out a loan
famous cities
things you build
places to go on vacation
things that are delivered
things that are hidden
things that roll

Items Needed: **20 balloons**

Group Size: **4 or more**

Format: **Pairs**
Group vs. Group

BLIND SPEAR FISHING

Blind Spear Fishing is probably one of our most superficially silly activities, but it turns out to be an excellent communication activity. Our processing time at the end is usually very lively because the action clearly shows clients the importance of direct, precise directions and the need for requesting clarification.

Procedure

The group is divided into pairs. One member of each team is blindfolded and given a "spear" (we find that coat hangers work just fine). The other member must verbally direct the blindfolded partner to a pool of fish. We use cardboard fish cutouts with rubber bands stapled to their noses, and stand them up by putting them between two large books. The sighted partner must verbally guide his teammate to catch a fish on his hook, turn around and walk a few feet to an awaiting bucket and drop it in. Typically, one person from each pair must catch two fish and then switch places with his partner. Sounds easy, huh? Try it! This one is also great for working on patience!

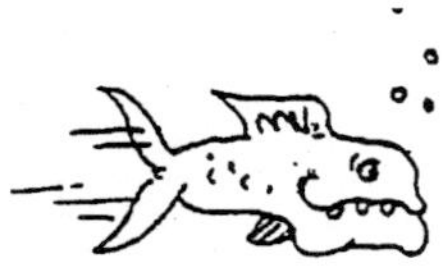

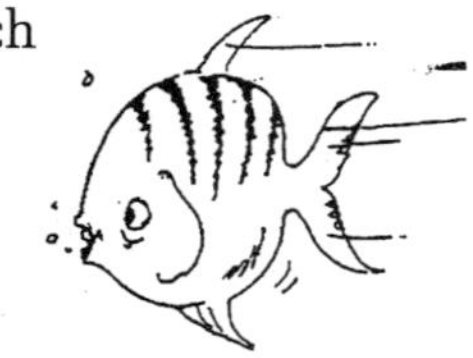

Items Needed: **blindfolds**
cardboard fish cutouts
rubber bands
basket
stack of books

Group Size: **4 or more**

Format: **Pairs**

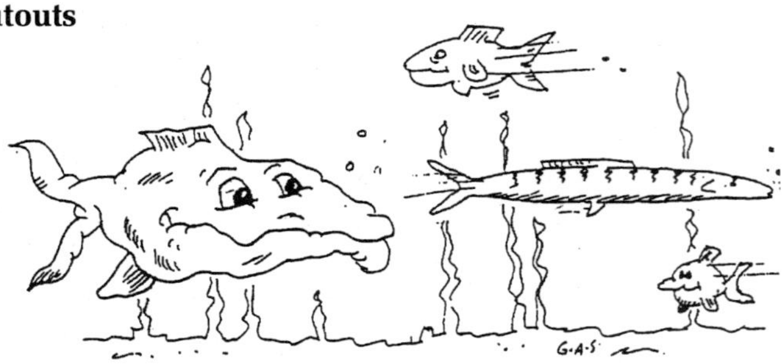

BODY BUILDING

Just what the name implies...kind of.

Body Building is like *Walkie Talkie Towers* in that it is a giant barrier game. Barrier activities are excellent communication tasks because they demand precise directions and detail-oriented questions, or they just won't work. Removing the barrier at the end provides a nice, concrete, visual picture of whether or not the group's communication was successful.

Procedure

Set up a large barrier — like a movable blackboard. Put half the group on one side and half the group on the other. One group needs to build something with their bodies and then explain to the other side how to create exactly the same thing. They can put an elbow on someone's shoulder, stick a finger in an ear, sit on a lap, anything that they are comfortable with. The barrier needs to be movable because each side ultimately needs to see what the other one looks like. Obviously, the people can't move because that would ruin their creation and there would be nothing to compare! In writing

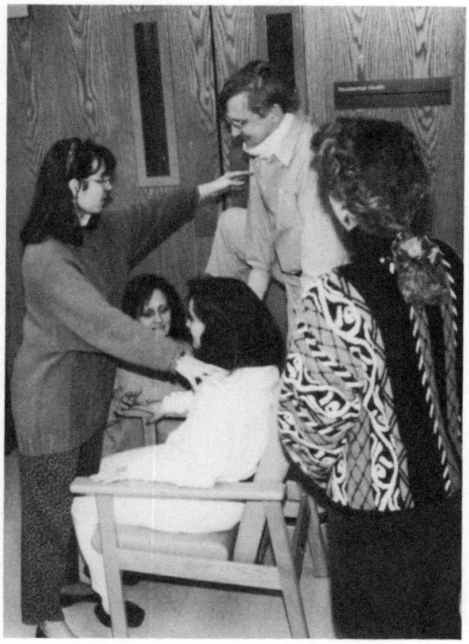

this, it occurs to me that it would be kind of interesting to see if the two sides could move their sculpture a few feet away from the barrier while still maintaining their shape. Let the sides exchange roles a few times, as time permits.

In order to get everyone talking, we ask that each person be the primary direction giver for the information that relates to his or her own body. If you are using *Body Building* for P.T. purposes, you can quietly tell the creating group that their building must somehow involve everyone standing on one leg, or doing a stretch, or anything else that will help to meet your physical goals.

Although you could do this activity with as little as one person per side, we have found that four per side works really well. We have listed this as a six person or more activity (adding up, you may have figured out, to just three per side). We are expecting that the leaders will join in to make up the difference.

Items Needed: **large barrier**

Group Size: **6 or more**

Format: **Group vs. Group**

BULLSEYE

Bullseye requires a bit of space. Outdoors is best, but a big room will work fine, too. The leaders should wear their running shoes because they'll get plenty of exercise chasing down beanbags to keep everyone supplied with ammo. Since half the group will be blindfolded, you'll also have to be aware of spotting needs.

Procedure

The group should be paired off. Draw a circle four feet in diameter on the ground in chalk or mark it off with rope. The circle should be big enough for half of the people to fit into and be able to move around each other. You'll need a bigger circle for more people, or for people using wheelchairs or walkers. Various sized receptacles or targets are placed outside the circle. These could include garbage pails, coffee cans, and pieces of cloth. These targets are placed at varying distances from the circle. One person from each pair (the shooter) stands inside the circle with a blindfold on and a supply of beanbags or other handy ammo. His partner (the aimer) gives him directions as to how to hit his bullseyes. The partners can also be responsible for spotting and keeping the shooters out of each others' way.

Points are given for each direct hit. Assign more points to harder targets. With post-it paper, indicate on each target the order in which it should be hit. For example, the garbage can might have 2 D on it. This means that the team following numbers aims at it second (2) and the team following letters aims at it fourth (D). If there are more than two teams, you can use different colors for each team's numbers (red team, blue team, green team). Ordering the targets adds one more degree of complexity for the teams, but mostly helps keep them out of each others' way. Remember to switch roles so everyone gets a chance to be an aimer and a shooter.

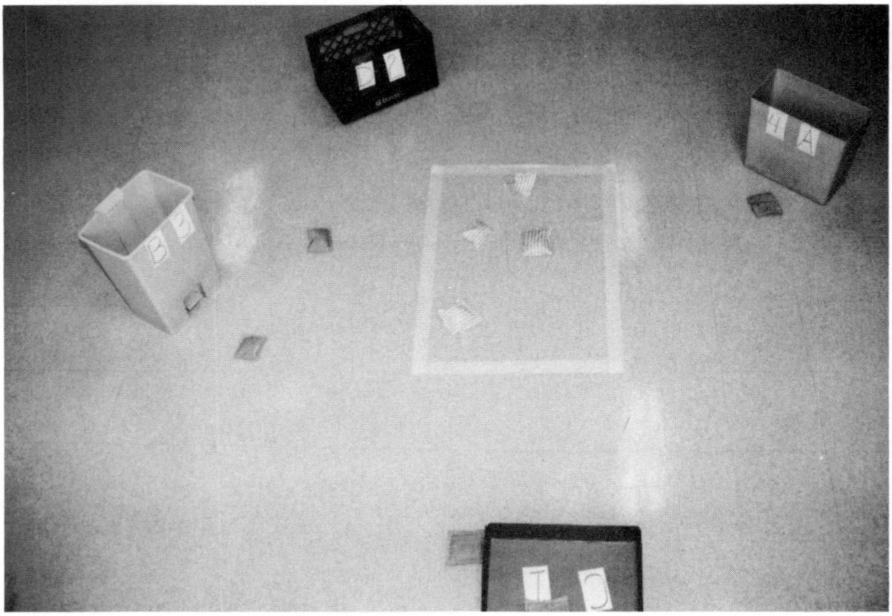

Processing topics might include: quality/precision of directions, frustration and relative demands of the two different roles.

Variations

If it is nice outside, use water balloons instead of beanbags for an extra touch of excitement. If getting the beanbags inside the targets is too difficult during the first round, allow points for just hitting any part of the target during the second round.

Items Needed: **several garbage cans**
buckets of varying sizes
pieces of cloth (additional targets)
blindfolds
beanbags

Group Size: **4 or more**

Format: **Pairs**

BULLSEYE II

You can easily move into *Bullseye II* if the group does well or tires quickly from *Bullseye I.* Transform the circle in *Bullseye I* into an actual bullseye. Assign varying points to the different rings. The format is the same in that there are aimers and shooters. This time, though, the shooters stand (blindfolded, of course) behind a line and shoot at the bullseye. The pairs can shoot from the same or different lines. The shooters should be blindfolded before the starting lines are made and then verbally guided to them so they do not know how far from the target they are. Multiple shooting lines can be drawn. Shooters can be guided from one line to another, with each line a different distance from the circle. Shooters take three throws from each line so they have a chance to modify their throws and aimers have an opportunity to modify their directions. Again, make sure aimers become shooters and vice versa.

Variation

Play on grass and substitute putting golf balls for throwing beanbags. Impose a time limit and use an unlimited number of golf balls or beanbags.

Items Needed: **tape or chalk (to make circles and starting lines)**
blindfolds
beanbags

Group Size: **4 or more**

Format: **Pairs**

BURGLARS AND LASERS

Use your imagination to create a vivid scenario for *Burglars and Lasers*. It might go like this: "You and your partner have just committed the perfect crime. You have stolen the Myopian Diamond from its perch in a British museum. But the police have sealed off your intended escape route and now your only way out is through a laser field. Your partner got through before the lasers were activated and she is the only one with the special laser finding glasses, so she must talk you through. You may not touch a laser with any part of your body. If you do, an alarm will sound and the police will know exactly where you are."

Procedure

Divide the group into pairs. Set up two rows of chairs about 5 feet apart and 14 feet in length. Wrap a rope around the legs of the chairs at just below knee height in a weblike fashion. Or outside, instead of chairs, you can use stakes normally used for roping off areas of grass. Each hole in the web should be big enough for a foot to fit in. These ropes are the lasers. A member of each team is selected to go first. The two who are up first stand side by side facing the web. They are blindfolded and their partner must talk them through the lasers. You should hear lots of directions, questions, and probably a "Watch out!" or two. When someone reaches the end of the laser field, he switches roles with his partner. Spotters can be used for those with poor balance or those who are afraid of falling. The use of spotters also increases trust between group members.

You can impose your own restrictions depending on the level of the group. For example, you can say that if someone touches a laser he must go back to the beginning or the team with the least alarm soundings wins, etc.

During your debrief, you might ask them what they needed to do in order to be successful. You might hear, "I really needed to concentrate, to listen carefully, to take small steps, to move slowly, to hold onto someone's shoulder for support, or to give lots of detail." Ask which role was more fun or frustrating. See what they might change about their communication or the way they moved if they were to do it again.

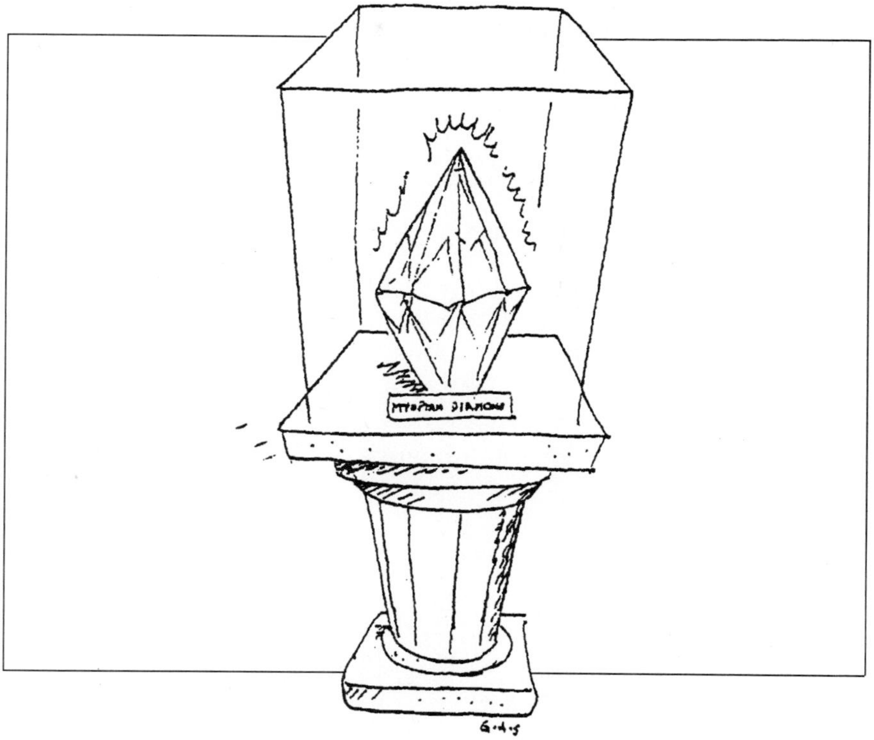

Modifications

For people in wheelchairs or with canes, walkers or simply poor balance, tape can be put directly on the floor to serve as lasers. The only thing that may not touch the lasers is a part of the body. Therefore, chairs can roll over them and walkers and canes can touch them and the lasers will not sound the alarm.

Items Needed: **chairs and 30 feet of rope or a roll of tape**
blindfolds

Group Size: **4 or more**

Format: **Pairs**

CHAIN REACTION

Chain Reaction is a good activity for problem-solving. Depending on how many elements you include and the level of your group, the *Chain Reaction* may be solved quickly, so be prepared with a backup activity or a variation of this one. The variation can simply involve different objects. You may want to take a few minutes and try to solve this yourself, first. You'll need to carefully choose the amount and size of items you give the group depending on the length of the table.

Procedure

Provide the group with a box of dominoes, two paper towel rolls, one block and a marble. At one end of a long table, stand an object on the edge that can easily be knocked over. We use an empty toilet tissue roll (they're cheap and we can get people to save them for us without too much prodding!). Put a starting line at the other end of the table a few inches in from the edge. The marble must be released from behind the starting line in order to start the *Chain Reaction*.

The object of the activity is to knock over the object at the end of the table via some sort of *Chain Reaction.* The marble must be simply released — not forcibly rolled or pushed. This means that they cannot simply push the marble across the table, hit the toilet paper roll and knock it over. That lacks imagination!

The only other rule is that the *Chain Reaction* cannot be a straight line; there must be at least one bend in it. Be sure not to give them enough dominoes to reach from the starting line to the final object. We are currently trying to think of some more objects to add so that we can use a longer table and add to the complexity, time and fun. See what you can come up with!

During the debrief you might discuss the relative contributions of each team member to the problem solving process. You can discuss the merits and weaknesses of the solution they developed and brainstorm alternatives.

Items Needed: **dominoes**
2 paper towel rolls
1 block

Group Size: **2 or more**

Format: **Group**

CHUTES AND 'LOONS

Chutes and 'Loons requires more hot air from the leaders than usual. That's because the "'loons" are actually balloons that need to be blown up beforehand. About 30 balloons are blown up and taped all over a wall, and a chute is placed nearby. This chute can be a large garbage can or bag or just a large piece of paper rolled to form a tube and taped to the wall with a bag on the end. It's most fun and challenging if the opening of the chute is only slightly larger than the 'loons.

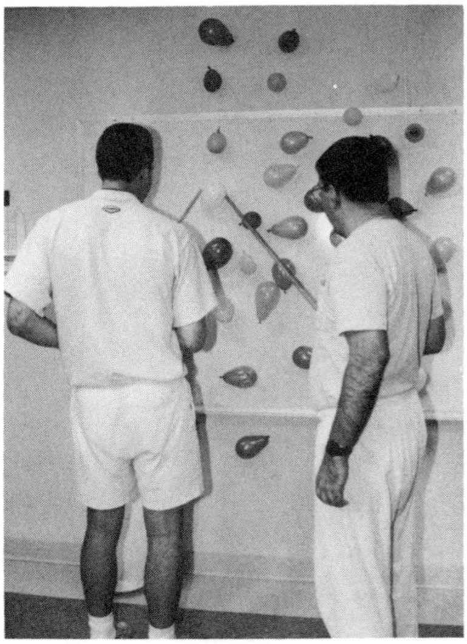

Procedure

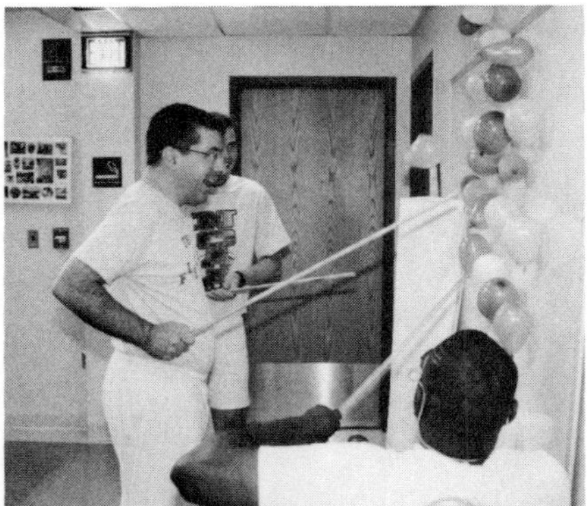

Members are paired off into teams. There should be as many chutes as there are teams. The object is for each team to get as many 'loons off the wall and into their chute as possible. The team with the most wins. Each 'loon must be put into the chute via a team effort. They may use any body parts they wish except their hands. That means that wrists, heads, noses, elbows, sides, knees and anything are fair game.

We have had a lot of success matching the more physically impaired clients with the more physically able. Though this activity emphasizes physical skills and communication, it also involves problem solving.

Variation 1

One pair came up with this variation when they misunderstood the directions. They took each new 'loon off the wall using a different body part. At various times, they were nose to nose, elbow to elbow and side by side. Even after we clarified the directions, they were having so much fun thinking of what to use next that they decided to keep on going. They lost, but they had fun doing it!

Variation 2

Each client is given a dowel (or stick or broom handle, etc.). The pairs must use their sticks to get the 'loons off the wall and into their chutes. This version is much more challenging and can lead to some frustration (which may be your goal). Keep the encouragement flowing and they are likely to make it through without turning their dowels against you! Keep in mind that this variation is not likely to work well with clients who are very ataxic. What you could do, though, is to substitute something a little less awkward for the 'loons (maybe like sponges or pieces of cloth) and use shorter dowels or tennis rackets.

Variation 3

This variation is good to throw at them as a time-filler if they happen to finish your first version quickly. Here, one member of each team has to get as many 'loons onto the other member as he can. 'Loons can go under chins and arms, in hands, between legs and anywhere else they can think of. We used this one to demonstrate to an upset girl in a wheelchair that her chair could actually be an asset. Because she had a lap and could hold both of her feet off the ground, she could hold more 'loons than anyone else and her team won. All the other teams ended up having their "holder" sit, too. She left that day with a big smile and a new outlook.

Items Needed:

30 balloons
large garbage can, bag, or large piece of paper rolled up to form a tube
dowels, broom handles or similar objects

Group Size: **4 or more**

Format:

Pairs
Group vs. Group

COBWEB

Cobweb is a flat version of PA's *Spider Web. Spider Web* is an excellent activity for planning ahead, problem solving, memory, flexible thinking and communication. In *Spider Web,* a rope web is suspended between two trees. The group must get everyone to the other side with no two people passing through the same hole. The physical lifting and mobility required are too demanding for our clients...so, we changed it.

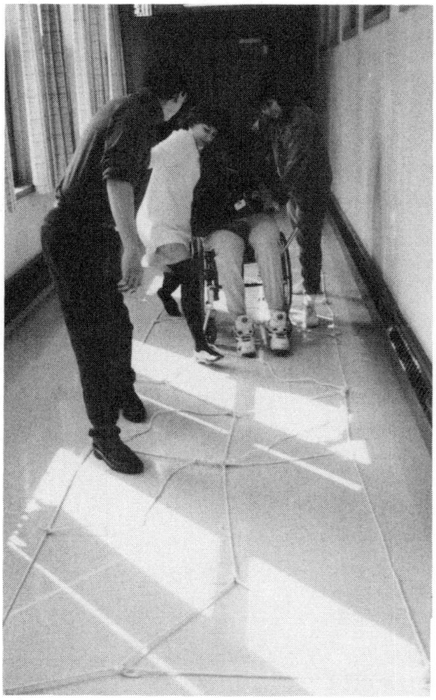

Procedure

In *Cobweb*, the web is laid out on the floor. It can be made out of tape placed directly on the floor or a rope can be taped into place on the floor. We are tired of getting tape off the floor, so we made ours out of rope, tying it into the shape of a cobweb. It took about two hours to make it initially, but now each time we want to use it we just pull it out of the closet, unroll it, tape it down and we are ready to go. Wheelchairs roll easily over the rope.

Like *Spider Web*, participants must not step into a hole if someone has already used it. They must walk from one end of the web to the other. If anyone touches the rope or steps in a "used" hole, the entire group must go back to the beginning. Unlike *Spider Web*, in *Cobweb* the group members will have to use more than one hole per person since they will be traveling the length of the web and not just going through it.

Remembering which holes have already been used is a big problem for our cognitively impaired clients. Sometimes we have provided them with checkers pieces to use as markers.

To emphasize planning ahead, you can have them plan their route entirely before anyone can take a step.

If you realize too late that there are not enough holes available for the number of people in your group, you can always add a rule in the middle. For instance, tell them that they can step into a hole someone else has used only if that person has moved two more holes beyond it. They should only go into the same person's spot once, though. This rule stops them from simply following each other down a single course.

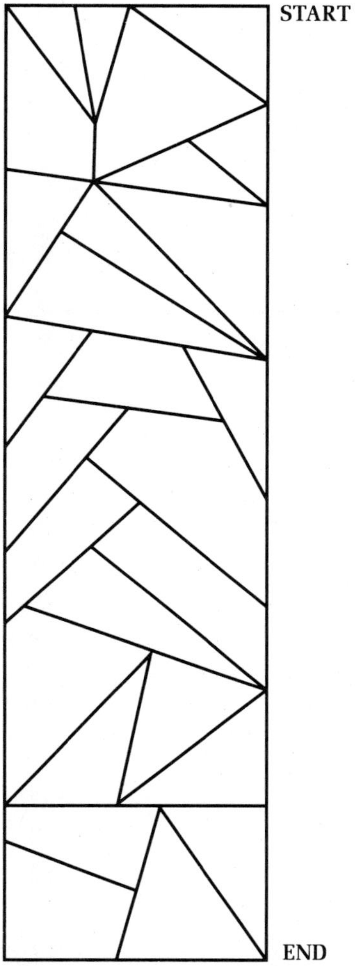

A person using a wheelchair, a walker, cane or crutches need only be concerned about where his feet go. If someone in a wheelchair cannot use his feet, he can be given a stick to touch the hole he is "in."

If your group solves *Cobweb* too quickly or you have too many holes and too few people, put some plastic spiders into some of the holes and have them try it without using those "occupied" holes.

Here is the layout that we use. It works well with five people.

Items Needed: **30–50 feet of rope made into a cobweb or a roll of tape**

Group Size: **4 or more (depends on number of holes in your cobweb)**

Format: **Group**

CROSSWORD

The objective of *Crossword* is to develop a crossword puzzle for another team to solve and then to solve the other team's puzzle. The challenge in *Crossword* typically comes more from creating your own puzzle than from solving the other team's. It takes planning, cooperation, reasoning, defining and visuo-spatial skills, just to name a few. Each of these areas then serves as a good topic for debriefing.

Procedure

Divide the group in half. Each group must create a crossword puzzle for the other group to solve. They need to draw it and come up with the clues. Remind them to give some thought to complexity. Their goal should not be to make it so hard that the other team will not be able to solve it. You can give them a theme or suggest they think of a theme. The theme can then be given to the other team or they can guess it after they have solved the puzzle.

Save the puzzles so that over time you will have enough for a crossword marathon on a rainy day. See who can solve the most in the time allowed.

Items Needed: **paper**
pencils

Group Size: **4 or more**

Format: **Group vs. Group**
Group
Pairs

DECODE THE CODE

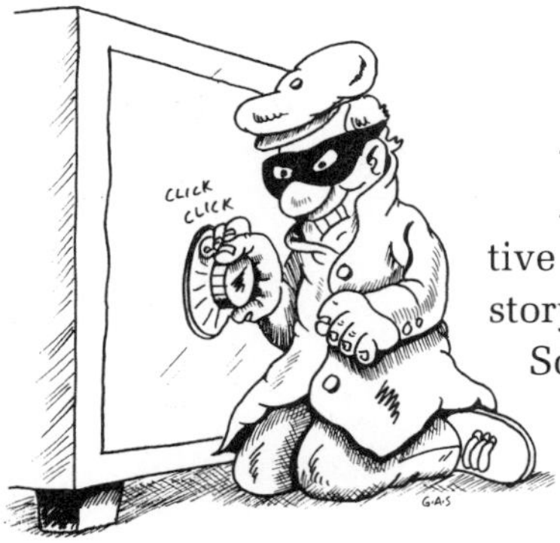

Here's a good activity to work on problem-solving, deductive reasoning skills, sequencing and organization. We wrote a story and coded each sentence of it onto separate slips of paper. Some of the codes include: writing the sentence backwards, using numbers instead of letters, writing in columns instead of rows and using no spaces in between words. You can simply photocopy the code pages and cut them into slips.

Procedure

First, the group must decipher each coded sentence and then organize them all into a story. As long as they can defend the reason for their sequence (if it differs from the original), we accept it. In fact, we frequently ask them to verbally defend their choices even if they do match. *Decode the Code* often takes two to three sessions, which is good because then they need to have some way of figuring out what they have already done when they come back to it. Notice that there is some awkward repetition of Bo's name in the story below. This is to help make it a little easier to solve. Use this story or write another one that's either simpler or more complex.

Modifications

If you have some people in the group that you know will have difficulty with this activity, pair them with someone with better skills and encourage that second person to help not tell. Often, our members work by themselves on some of the codes. That's okay because there are some things; i.e., figuring out which codes have already been solved and which haven't, that they must discuss as a group. It helps the group to see how their individual work ties into the whole. We once had a group whose members, working as individuals in isolation, were each solving codes and then placing them back into a central pile. They kept resolving each other's codes until someone realized what was going on. We had great content for debriefing that day!

If your group will have too much difficulty solving the codes, eliminate them and just have them put the story in order. Or, change all of the sentences to one type of code. Help them solve the first one and then let them use that concept to solve the rest. If putting the story in order would be too hard, let them solve the codes in order or number the coded slips.

The Story

Once upon a time in a land very far away lived a fair-skinned, freckle-faced boy and his green and yellow parrot. The boy's name was Bo and the parrot's name was Bart. No one knows how Bart got his name but 10 year old Bo. It happened on a warm spring day at the end of May. Bo was sitting high above the green pastures and colorful aromatic gardens on an ancient stone fence which surrounded the mansion in which Bo lived with his family. Bo was gazing up into the sky wondering what it would be like if he were able to fly. All of a sudden he heard the footsteps of someone walking toward him. He looked down. He could not believe his eyes. The figure below him was one that he had never seen before. He or she was about three feet tall. The head was oddly shaped with three eyes and a tiny mouth. This alien creature was trying to communicate with Bo. Bo didn't know whether to be frightened or elated. Curiosity got the better of Bo. He jumped down off the fence and said, "Hello, my name is Bo." The alien responded with a message unintelligible to the human ear. Bo attempted to communicate once more, but the alien fled before Bo could finish his sentence. Seconds later, something caught his eye in the grass where the alien once stood. There in the grass he found a tiny green and yellow parrot. The strange alien creature must have left this bird behind. "Maybe that's what he was trying to tell me," said Bo outloud. "I guess I'll call you Bart," said Bo to his new friend. "I think that's what the alien was saying to me," he said. Bo began to head for home, thinking about all that had happened. It was on his way home that he decided that he had better not ever tell anyone how Bart got his name.

Codes

The following codes are in order, so remember to mix them up if you want to make it more difficult.

15, 14, 3, 5   21, 16, 15, 14   1   20, 9, 13, 5   9, 14   1   12, 1, 14, 4   22, 5, 18, 25
6, 1, 18   1, 23, 1, 25   12, 9, 22, 5, 4   1   6, 1, 9, 18   19, 11, 9, 14, 14, 5, 4
6, 18, 5, 3, 11, 12, 5   6, 1, 3, 5, 4   2, 15, 25   1, 14, 4   8, 9, 19   7, 18, 5, 5, 14
1, 14, 4   25, 5, 12, 12, 15, 23   16, 1, 18, 18, 15, 20

TRAB SAW EMAN S'TORRAP EHT DNA OB SAW EMAN S'YOB EHT

NU UNI KNUWS HUW BERT GUT HOS NEMI BAT TIN YIER
ULD BU

YAM FO DNE EHT TA YAD GNIRPS MRAW A NO DENEPPAH TI

BOWASSITTINGHIGHABOVETHEGREENPASTURESANDCOLORFULARO
MATICGARDENSONANANCIENTSTONEFENCEWHICHSURROUNDEDTHE
MANSIONINWHICHBOLIVEDWITHHISFAMILY

2, 15,   23, 1, 19   7, 1, 26, 9, 14, 7   21, 16   9, 14, 20, 15   20, 8, 5   19, 11, 25
23, 15, 14, 4, 5, 18, 9, 14, 7   23, 8, 1, 20   9, 20   23, 15, 21, 12, 4   2, 5   12, 9, 11, 5
9, 6   8, 5   23, 5, 18, 5   1, 2, 12, 5   20, 15   6, 12, 25

ALLOFASUDDENHEHEARDTHEFOOTSTEPSOFSOMEONEWALKINGTOWAR
DHIM

NWODDEKOOLEH

SEYE SIH EVEILEB TON DLUOC EH

20, 8, 5   6, 9, 7, 21, 18, 5   2, 5, 12, 15, 23   8, 9, 13   23, 1, 19   15, 14, 5
20, 8, 1, 20   8, 5   8, 1, 4   14, 5, 22, 5, 18   19, 5, 5, 14   2, 5, 6, 15, 5

LLATTEEFEERHTTUOBASAWEHSROEH

T	D	D	P	H	E	D	M
H	W	L	E	T	Y	A	O
E	A	Y	D	H	E	T	U
H	S	S	W	R	S	I	T
E	O	H	I	E	A	N	H
A	D	A	T	E	N	Y	

T	A	N	A	E	T	N	C	U	A	I	O
H	L	C	T	W	R	G	O	N	T	T	
I	I	R	U	A	Y	T	M	I	E	H	
S	E	E	R	S	I	O	M	C	W	B	

2	14	23	8	2	7	14	12
15	20	23	5	5	8	4	1
4	11	8	18	6	20	15	20
9	14	5	20	18	5	18	5
4	15	20	15	9	5	5	4

OBFORETTEBEHTTOGYTISOIRUC

HEJUMPEDDOWNOFFTHEFENCEANDSAID"HELLOMYNAMEISBO"

T	I	S	E	H	S	N	L	B	T	M	R
H	E	P	D	A	A	I	L	L	H	A	
E	N	O	W	M	G	N	I	E	E	N	
A	R	N	I	E	E	T	G	T	H	E	
L	E	D	T	S	U	E	I	O	U	A	

OB DETPMETTA OT ETACINUMMOC ECNO TUB EHT NEILA

DELF EROFEB OB DLUOC HSINIF SIH ECNETNES

O	O	H	S	T	I	C	M	L	S
D	N	E	W	H	S	A	E	A	E
	C	A	H	E	E	U	T	T	C
	E	L	E	G	Y	G	H	E	O
	S	I	R	R	E	H	I	R	N
	T	E	E	A	I	T	N	S	D
	O	N	T	S	N	H	G	O	S

TORRAPWOLLEYDNANEERGYNITADNUOFEHSSARGEHTNIEREHT

EHT EGNARTS NEILA ERUTAERC TSUM EVAH TFEL SIHT DRIB DNIHEB

"MAYBETHATSWHATHEWASTRYINGTOTELLME"BOSAIDOUTLOUD DNEIRFWENSIHOTOBDIAS"TRABUOYLLACLLISSEUGI"

"I THINK THAT'S WHAT THE ALIEN WAS SAYING TO ME," HE SAID

B	A	E	R	T	I	O	L	H	P	N
O	N	A	H	H	N	U	T	A	P	E
B	T	D	O	I	G	T	H	D	E	D
E	O	F	M	N	A	A	A	H	N	
G	H	O	E	K	B	L	T	A	E	

OT WES UN HOS WEY HUMI THET HI DICODID THET HI HED

BITTIR NUT IVIR TILL ENYUNI HUW BERT GUT HOS NEMI

Items Needed: clues on separate slips of paper
pencils
extra paper

Group Size: 2 or more

Format: Group

DRAWING RELAY

More blindfolding and great fun, too! If you haven't already done it, go back and read the safety notes about blindfolding in Chapter Three. *Drawing Relay* is a good activity to use for groups that believe their communication is precise but who, in your estimation, are really having some difficulties. *Drawing Relay* will demand accurate communication and will concretely show when it has broken down. Be prepared for some frustration on the part of the art directors (see below).

Procedure

Divide the group into two teams. Everyone is blindfolded except for one person from each team. This person, the art director, is given a card with a drawing on it. Both art directors have the same objects on their cards. The art directors verbally direct one person at a time from their team to draw part of the picture on a blackboard. Their other blindfolded team members are sitting down a couple of feet from the board. When the first person is done drawing, the art director tells him how to get back to his seat and then verbally guides the next person to the board to draw the next part of the picture. The art directors must only give verbal directions. They cannot physically touch the person's hand in any way. Keep rotating through all the team members until all parts of the picture are drawn.

When each team is finished they can take off their blindfolds and look at the finished product. Good Grief! This is the best part. Take some time to talk about what they will change about their communication before they put the blindfolds back on for round two.

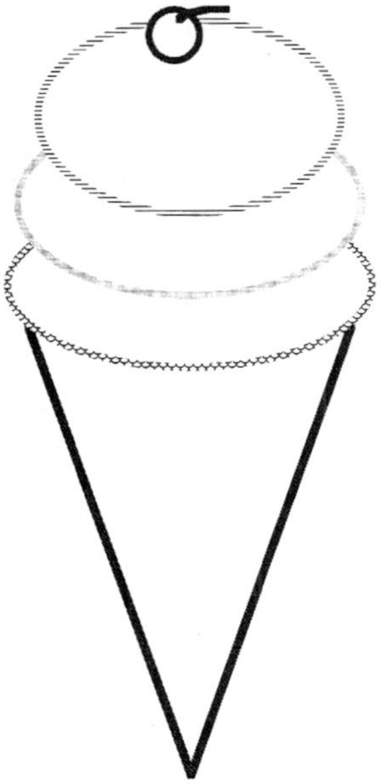

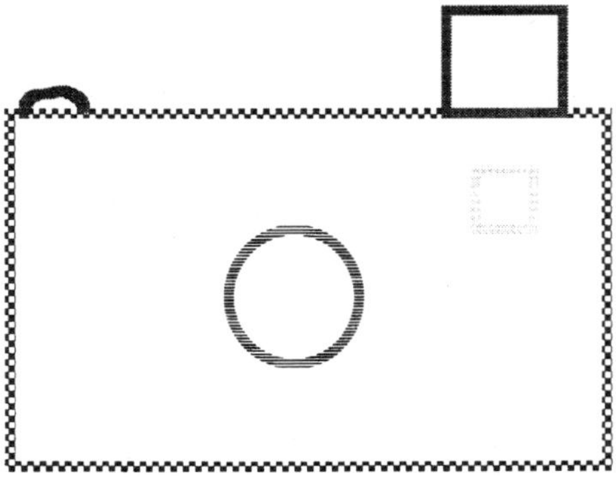

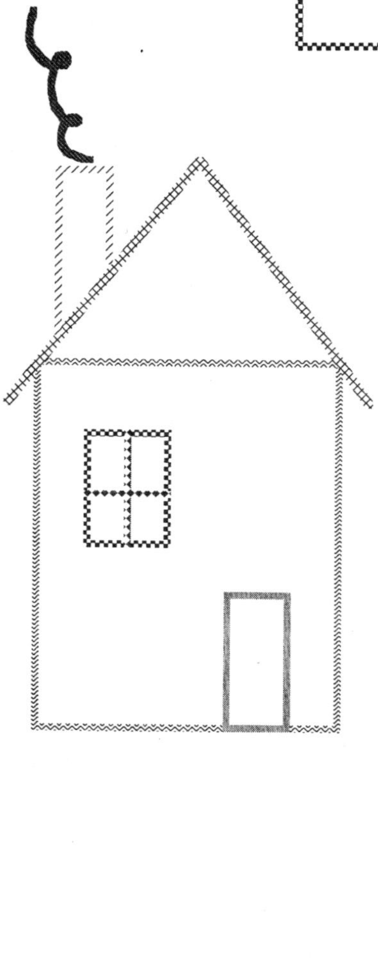

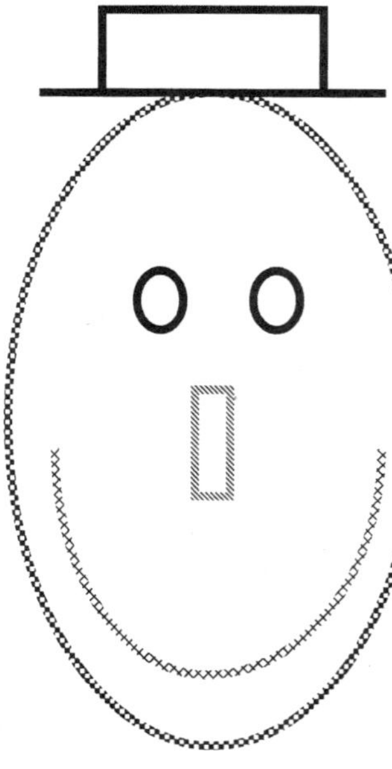

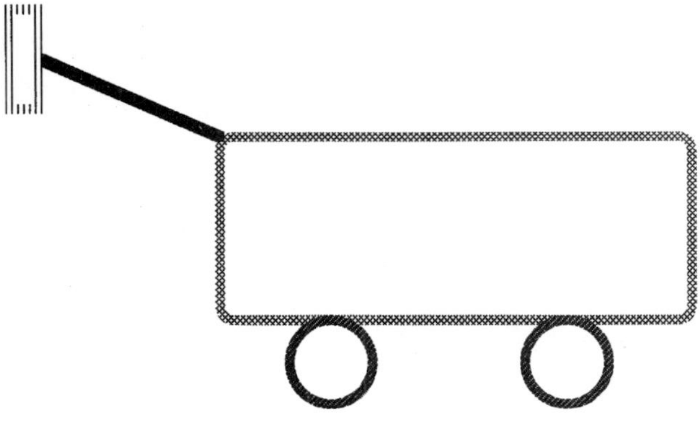

Keep the drawings simple. You may use ours or create your own. Notice that the lines of the different portions of the drawings are different from each other. Each change in print style represents a different drawer. We put the drawings on cardboard or index cards and draw each part with a different color.

Drawing Relay works on trust, auditory comprehension, verbal expression and fine motor skills.

Modifications

Instead of using a blackboard, you can do the *Drawing Relay* on a table top with a piece of paper. Then simply pass the paper to each new person. This would be an appropriate modification for use with people who would have difficulty reaching the board, would have difficulty walking up to the board while blindfolded, or would need their arm stabilized on the table top in order to draw.

Items Needed:

drawings
blindfolds
chalk
blackboard

Group Size: **6 or more**

Format: **Group vs. Group**

DRESSING RELAY

The *Dressing Relay* is great fun — and a great communication exercise, too. On several occasions, we've had individuals in the group who view themselves as very adult, very serious, and too proper to have fun. We debated whether or not to do *Dressing Relay* because it entails dressing up and looking, well, goofy. In the end, we've always been pleasantly surprised with the clients' reactions. At the finish of the activity, gather around and take a group picture — guaranteed to bring a smile if nothing else has.

Procedure

Gather all the funny clothes you can find including hats, aprons, cooking mitts, large gardening gloves, boots, pants, and shirts. Then spread them out in a large open area. Divide the group into pairs. Blindfold one member of each pair and give the other a list of specific clothes. At the start, the one with the list verbally guides the other to the first piece of clothing on the list and gets him to put it on without using its name. For example, for an apron he might say, "Feel for two strings and tie them around your waist."

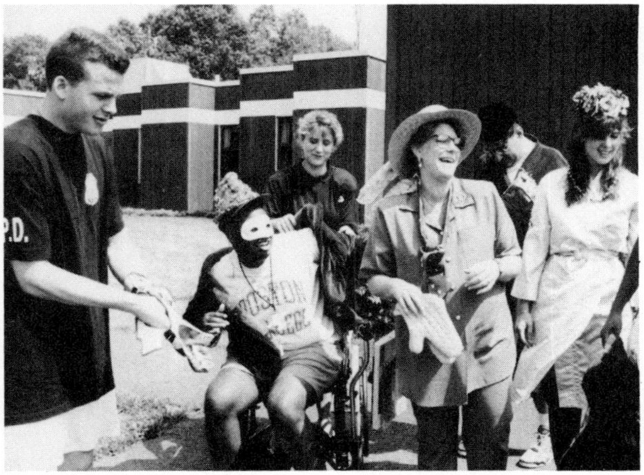

As soon as the first member of the pair has all the clothes on from the list, they trade roles and are given a new list. The first one must stay dressed in these clothes until the end. This activity always provokes a lot of laughter and playful kidding. It's also great for working on basic direction giving and receiving.

Modifications

Hey, O.T.'s and P.T.'s — how about using the *Dressing Relay* for a fun, nontraditional approach to working on actual dressing skills with physically impaired clients? You could leave off the blindfolds and focus on using adaptive equipment and procedures. Just use bigger clothes that will fit over street clothes.

Vocational therapists could use a combination of appropriate (ties, jackets, etc.) and inappropriate clothing (ripped jeans, dirty shirts, etc.) and have each client get his partner to dress only in the clothing appropriate for his type of work. The debriefing part of the session could revolve around how to dress for the workplace.

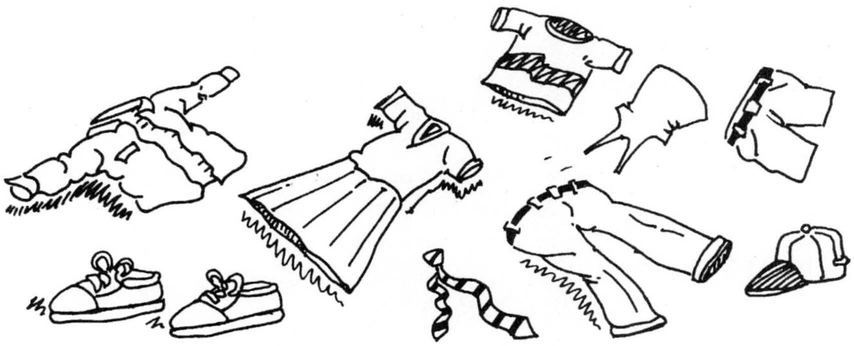

Items Needed: **hats**
aprons
cooking mitts
gardening gloves
boots
pants
shirts
coats
vests
scarves

Group Size: **4 or more**

Format: **Pairs**

FILLET OF SOLE

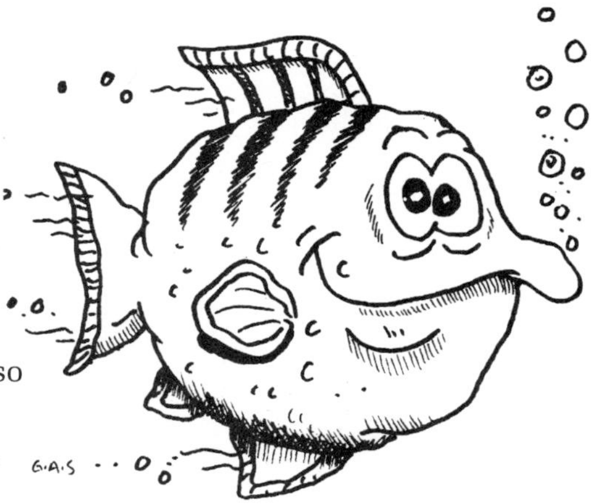

Fillet of Sole is a big challenge for clients with cognitive deficits. It taxes their ability to maintain a mental set and to determine relevant versus irrelevant information. It also places heavy demands on verbal reasoning and verbal expression.

Procedure

The group is given the problem statement: *How to Prepare Fillet of Sole*. This statement can be made verbally, written on the board or written on an index card and put on the table. Then a pile of cards with the "sideline" statements below written on them are divided evenly among the group members. Their goal is to decide as a group whether each sideline relates to the problem statement. Some will be obvious, but others will be much more subtle. Our head injured groups have the most difficulty with sidelines that are true and on the subject of fish, but don't really have anything to do with how to prepare it. An example is "Fish is low in cholesterol." They will say, "Yes, I know that's true," and the card will get stacked in the relevant pile without further thought. Some groups do not think to create relevant and irrelevant piles. They go through each person's cards and make their decisions and then have to go back through them all over again at the end when we ask them to tell us all the relevant sidelines.

Be sure to have them defend their choices at the end. Make sure that everyone can explain their rationale. Challenge both right and wrong answers. As long as they can come up with a plausible defense for a sideline to be included in either pile, accept it. But if it is just completely wrong, point out the error in their reasoning.

Our sidelines are listed below. They can easily be copied onto index cards once and then used over and over again.

Sidelines:

Fish is low in cholesterol.
For healthy soles, see your podiatrist.
After defrosting, dip fish in egg mixture, flour and place in a skillet.
Your soul continues on after you die.
Beware of bones when eating your fillet of sole.
Your soles may ache after a long walk along a river.
Lightly sprinkle with paprika.
Some cultures believe that the eyes are windows to the soul.
Broil the fillet of sole for 10 minutes.
Slice 2 onions and place over fish before cooking.
Prepare wine sauce 15 minutes ahead of time.
Sole is delicious buttered and lightly fried.
Rinse your sole under warm water.
Burger Palace fries their fillet of sole and serves it on a bun.
Fish can be baked and served over ice.
Sole is my favorite dish.
I don't like fish, so I wouldn't prepare it.

Items Needed: **problem statements and sidelines printed on index cards**

Group Size: **2 or more**

Format: **Group**

FOWL PLAY

The poultry pluckers are coming! The poultry pluckers are coming! And your somewhat fearless leader is a chicken — literally! You must work together to get the chicken to the other side of your island where it is safe. Because he is your fearless leader, the chicken must be treated with the utmost respect at all times!

Procedure

All you will need for this activity is a rope approximately 35 feet long, a rubber chicken (or any stuffed animal) and a big enough box to accommodate your prized poultry. Working as a group, the clients must transport their cherished mascot from one side of an island to the other. They can only use what you have already given them (the box and the rope).

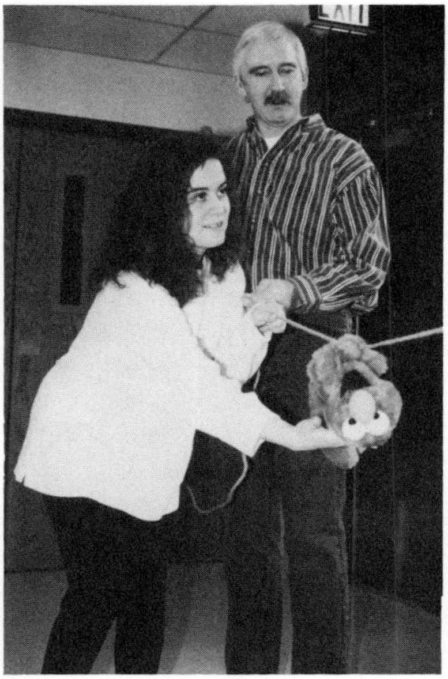

The problem is that the chicken must go directly across the island, over sacred ground, but the group members can only skirt around the outside. Show them a narrow space about 15 feet long that will serve as the middle of the island where they dare not tread. If it helps, mark off the area with tape, chalk or rope. They may not do anything along the long sides to aid in the solution. For example, they may not hold the chicken in their hands over the sacred ground while walking along the sides. They can only move themselves along the sides, like if they decide they want more people on one end or the other.

Because the chicken is such a valued member of the small island's inner circle, he cannot be thrown, kicked or rolled to the other side of the island. He also may not be tied up in an undignified way. We'll leave the interpretation of "undignified" up to you. The definition can vary depending on how difficult or easy a time they are having. He may not touch the middle portion of the island, nor should the box or rope. Instead he must be transported above it. Reiterate several times, especially if you see any undignified handling, that the chicken must be handled with the utmost respect at all times!

There are several possible solutions to *Fowl Play.* If the group solves it quickly, you can challenge them to challenge their divergent thinking skills and come up with another solution. Often this second solution is more difficult to think of than the first, especially with cognitively rigid clients.

One other suggestion: have a camera ready because it's a riot to see the mascot being transported across the inner territory. Surely it's a sight you'll want to capture for posterity.

Possible Solutions

Spend a few minutes thinking before you read on.
That way you'll get an idea about what your group is in for.

1) If the rope is long enough, they can put the chicken in the box; send one end of the rope across sacred ground to some awaiting team members; pass the rope across the top of the open box; close the lid, folding in the flaps; lift the rope, which should lift the box; and let the rope out while the other side pulls it toward them. Variations on this theme include having the chicken stick partially out of the box or, trickier still, having him ride on top.
2) If the rope is shorter, they can try this same approach, but have one end lower their rope while the other end raises theirs so the box will slide along it. The box doesn't always slide that well, so they might instead try option #3.
3) Poke holes in opposite sides of the box, run the ropes through and slide the box along the rope as above.
4) Eliminate the box and tie the chicken up in a dignified way. We usually accept a knot around its upper body as dignified. Of course, the chicken must remain upright the entire way across. We do not allow them to tie its legs into a loop, pass the rope through and then slide it upside down to the awaiting teammates. Although this is unacceptable for us, you can decide what's acceptable in your neck of the woods. By the way, no tying the rope around the chicken's neck, either!

We've seen attempts to send either the box and chicken or just the chicken across the sacred territory on top of the rope — just sliding along the top of a very taut rope — but we've never seen it done successfully ...yet!

As we've said above, encourage divergent thinking if the group solves it quickly. If you gave them a long rope initially, say, "shoot, that wasn't the sacred rope. The chicken needs to be transported with *this* rope." Pull out a shorter one and have the group try again. In the debrief, be sure to recognize their ability to think of an alternate solution.

Items Needed: **35 foot rope**
rubber chicken (or whatever you choose your sacred leader to be)
big box

Group Size: **4 or more**

Format: **Group**

GAMEMASTER

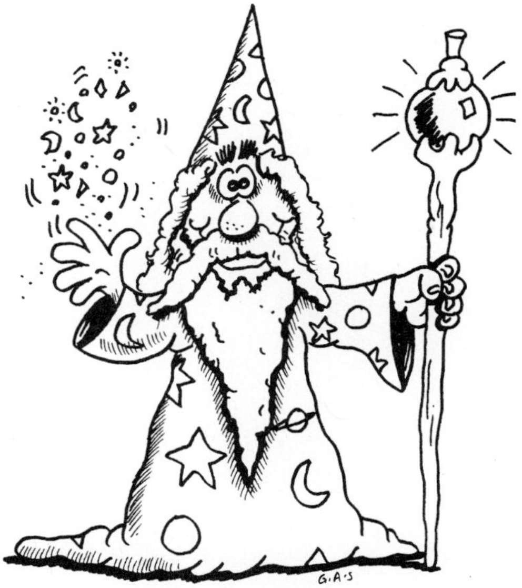

With every new group of clients, we are inevitably asked (with frightening similarity), "What are you going to do to us to-day?!" and, "How late did you stay up thinking of this one?!" Luckily, there's always a glimmer of eager anticipation behind their questions. We typically answer something like, "Ooh, this is a good one! We were on the phone until three in the morning. I'm a little tired this morning. Does it show?"

Gamemaster is their opportunity to get back at us. In *Gamemaster* they create the game. As long as it fits certain parameters, we'll try it. Our parameters may be different from yours. Activities for our group must somehow involve communication and be challenging, but safe, for the members.

We have never actually set this as the main activity for the session because it is very difficult. We have had individuals who have been ready for the challenge, but never an entire group. We have offered this feat to some higher level individuals during their final days in the group, but no one has ever come up with an idea.

Variation:

We just said that we've never done *Gamemaster* because we've never had a group cognitively ready for it. But, of course, we do have a modified version that we have used! The problem for our clients is that the *Gamemaster* above does not have enough structure. So, we give them structure. Following some of the activities, we have them think of some variations, or we challenge them to come up with a new activity based on the same structure. For instance, if *Fillet of Sole* ends early, we might have them think of another main statement and sidelines. They can also think of some additional license plates for *Who's Driving That Car?* and *Road Trip*. For *Decode the Code*, you can give two groups newspaper stories of equal complexity, have them code the stories and then switch with the other group and solve them.

Items Needed: **whatever they decide they need**

Group Size: **1 or more**

Format: **Group**

GET IT TOGETHER

Oh no! Blindfolded again?! Not necessarily.

Get it Together is good for working on stereognosis (recognizing objects by touch), inductive (part to whole) reasoning, multimodal processing, visualization, memory, verbal expression and attention to detail. All of these areas are then fair game for processing. It may help to have the group discuss what *Get It Together* is working on after you give the instructions during the brief.

Procedure

Sitting in a circle, each person is either blindfolded or trusted to keep his or her eyes closed or given a box they can reach into but not see into. Without seeing it, each person reaches into the box and picks out an item. Talking to each other, the group tries to decide what the pieces would make if they were assembled. They cannot show their piece to someone else or let them touch it. Random guessing is discouraged by subtracting a point for every incorrect guess. Two points are given for every correct guess. Once the entire group comes to a decision, the leader tells them yes or no and changes the score accordingly. It is fine if someone has two objects or has no objects in some rounds depending on the number of parts each whole item has. If everyone is adequately describing what they are holding, even someone without a piece should be able to participate.

If the group absolutely has no idea what the object is and everyone has described their piece, have each person pass their piece to the person to their right and let the discussion continue. They can keep going until they either guess it correctly or get their own piece back. If it is appropriate for the group, they can assemble the object after they have guessed it.

If you think the group will react negatively to being blindfolded, you can have everyone push their chairs in close to the table and pass the box underneath the table as they select their pieces. Keep in mind that having their eyes open, they will be more likely to take turns talking and they will know more readily that someone was listening when they spoke (through eye contact).

Possibilities

- Toy car
- Barbie doll
- Pen
- Wok and chopsticks
- Dustbuster
- Bicycle pump
- Shirt pieces
- Watch
- Clock
- Electric pencil sharpener and pencil

Items Needed **box**
any of the items desired above in the Possibilities list

Group Size: **3 or more**

Format: **Group**

GET OUTA TOWN

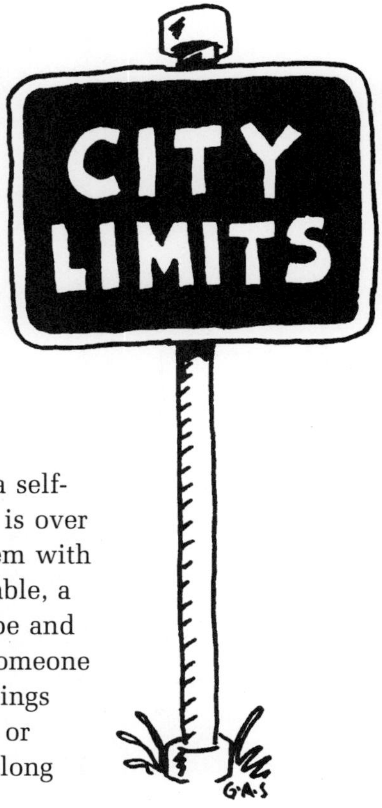

Get Outa Town is for groups that can handle less structure. Its primary emphasis is on how the group goes about applying their own structure or developing a plan. The leaders can always add more structure or provide more cueing if it becomes evident that the group needs it.

Procedure

The group's objective is to design a self-sufficient town. The next closest town is over one-hundred miles away. We leave them with a large piece of paper the size of the table, a pile of construction paper, scissors, tape and markers. The only stipulation is that someone else must be able to figure out what things are, so the clients need to make a key, or label the buildings or something else along those lines. Then just let them go.

Debriefing

During the debrief, talk about why the group included what they did and why other things were not included. For instance, "What made you decide to include a train station? Why don't you have a food store?" Have them talk about how they went about developing a plan. Was it random? Did they just put things in when they thought of them? Or was there some grander plan regarding where things were in relation to others? Would they change this planning process if they were to do it again? How easily could someone use their key or labels if they were just coming into the group? Have them discuss a good name for the town. If they had to elect city officials based on their performance, who would get what job? We tend not to make judgments about any of the group's decisions. Our goal is just for them to be able to verbally defend their choices and think things through.

Items Needed:

one very large piece of paper (the size of the table)
construction paper
scissors
tape
markers
pencils

Group Size: **2 or more**

Format: **Group**

HOW TO TREAT A COLD

How to Treat a Cold is the same as *Fillet of Sole*, but with a different problem statement and sidelines. This second version is good for assessing carryover of skills. *How to Treat a Cold* has almost twice as many sidelines. Use as many as you need.

Problem Statement: **How to Treat a Cold**

Sidelines:

Drink plenty of liquids.
Take aspirin for your aches and pains.
When it gets cold, ice will freeze.
Get plenty of rest.
Its no fun to have a cold.
Colds can stop you from going to work.
Take a cold reliever that lists your specific symptoms.
Alaska is very cold most of the year.
See your doctor if the symptoms do not go away.
You will catch a cold if you drink from a sick person's cup.
Many cold relievers contain alcohol.
Cold weather may cause hypothermia.
Treat body aches with warm compresses.
Throat lozenges may help.
Some cold relievers may make you drowsy.
Be sure to follow the directions on the medication carefully.
Your nose may run if you have a cold.
Chicken soup is good on a cold day.
Prevent a cold by staying dry in cold weather.
Orange juice is good for a cold.
Chicken soup is said to be good for fighting a cold.

Orange juice contains lots of vitamin C.
Hot chocolate is good on a cold day.
Run the heat a little higher than you normally would.
Take extra vitamin C.
Don't push yourself too hard.
Some cold relievers are very expensive.
Smoke may irritate your nasal passages.
Stay home from work.
Nasal sprays can help stop a runny nose.

Variations

You may decide to make up your own problem statement and sidelines. It helps to use a word or phase that can be interpreted in several different ways like "sole". This new activity can be used to assess generalization of skills. Below are some possible problem statements. Just come up with some sidelines and you are ready to go.

Problem Statements:

How To Board A Plane
How To Plant A Rose Bush
How To Inflate A Beach Ball
How To Get Rid Of A Fly
How To Stay Cool In A Heat Wave
Why Fall Is A Good Time Of Year
How To Stay On The Balance Beam
How To Iron A Silk Shirt
What To Do In Case Of A Fire
How To Tell When Fruit Is Fresh
How To Build A Rock Wall

Group size: **3 or more**

Format: **Group**

IS IT?

Our format for *Is It?* is group versus group because competition has never been an issue for our groups when we have done this activity. That might be because the teams have different roles at any one time so they are not directly competing to be the first or the best. In fact, the team that has the answer usually ends up asking if they can help the other team and give them clues. So, the teams actually become pretty supportive of each other.

Procedure

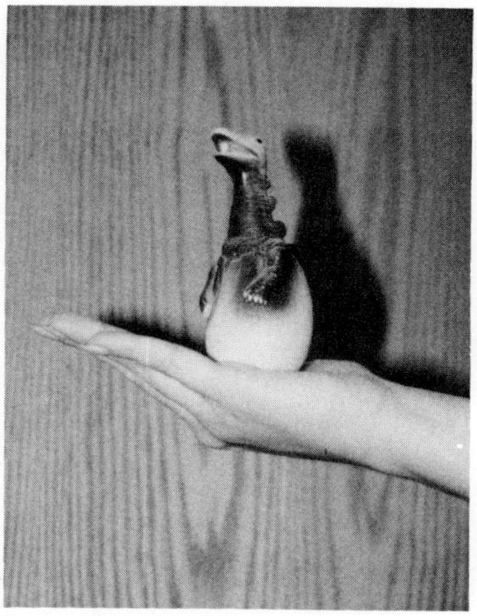

Divide the group into two teams. Give Team A three objects that they must hide outside the room. Give them some limits on what areas they can use; i.e., from the cafeteria to the fire exit and not in any treatment rooms, and how long they have to hide the objects; i.e., be back in five minutes. We like using odd objects — like maybe a Troll or a toy dinosaur. When Team A returns from hiding the objects, Team B must find them. In order to locate these objects, they can only ask Team A questions — they cannot go looking for them. They may ask as many questions as they need to. However, the questions can only elicit yes/no answers. Once the item locations are determined, the group can then go get them — if they can remember where they are! Our clients often need to be cued to take notes, or at least given subtle reminders that they will need to remember the information in order to find the items. As they find them, they should hide them somewhere else and then return to the room and give Team A a chance to ask the questions.

When you process what happened in *Is It?*, talk about the role of visualization and visual memory, the need for taking notes to remember the information gathered, and differences between the two roles of information givers and object finders.

Variations

Limit the number of questions asked. Have the questions answered only through facial expressions, and *no* head-nodding or speaking.

Items Needed: **3 odd objects**

Group Size: **4 or more**

Format: **Group vs. Group**

JUNKYARD SWING

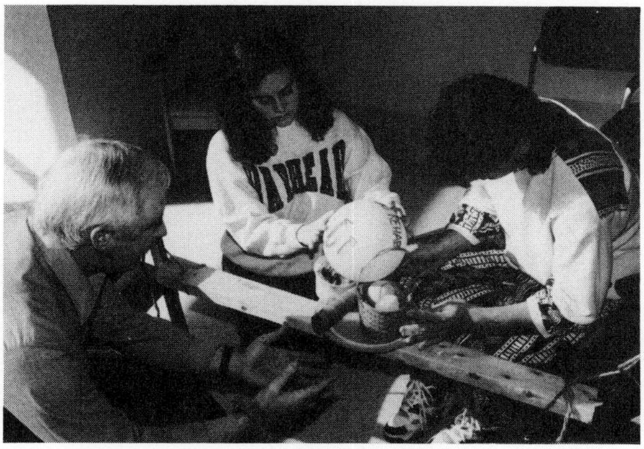

This activity is similar in basic concept to *Pile-On,* so it is a good one to assess generalization. *Junkyard Swing* does take a few props, but outside of the necessary rope, 2" x 4" board, and chairs, it doesn't matter what you use. Have some fun with the objects you choose. Your debrief might focus on planning, group interaction style, and the roles of the individuals.

Procedure

Two chairs are placed back to back, about six feet apart. A two-foot (or so) section of wood (2x4 is good) is suspended long ways between them by rope. So, you should have two pieces of rope tied to the ends of a 2x4 and then tied to the backs of two chairs, ending up with the 2x4 suspended one to two feet above the ground. The group is given a pile of random objects and told that they must get all of those things onto the wood without using or touching the support ropes. They can't hold or steady the wood in any way.

They cannot take something off once it has been placed on the wood. This rule is to encourage planning without actually having to say, "plan ahead!" If an object falls into the abyss below, the group must start all over. In the spirit of the Adventure Wave, though, this need to start over can be reframed as a positive opportunity to learn from what they just did wrong and to try a new plan. There is always another chance to succeed. If, on the other hand, something falls off and someone catches it before it actually touches the floor (becomes lost in the abyss), they can continue from where they are. This rule is to encourage everyone to be on the alert at all times.

The first time we did *Junkyard Swing,* the group finished very quickly because of some good problem solving. They decided to build on the floor first, to eliminate the need to worry about and deal with the wood swinging. We decided not to take this option away from them because we thought it was a great idea. We had never pictured-solving it in this way. Sometimes the most obvious things elude us! This left us with the activity completed and 30 minutes to go! If you'd like, you can take this option away ahead of time by telling them that all assembly must occur on the wood.

Modification

Luckily we had a modification ready to go. We allowed them to choose one item to take out of their pile. This decision forced a nice discussion and some good reasoning. Once they eliminated the object we added two more. One was a very small water balloon and the other was a light; i.e., fake volleyball. Again, we got something we did not anticipate. The ball really made their pile top-heavy and it would not stay balanced once it was on the wood, despite the fact that it was stable on the ground. This new problem made them have to completely rethink things. Time ran out before they were done and we had a great debrief.

What happened to us underscores the need for leaders to go into activities prepared for things to go wrong or to go quickly. Be prepared with another way to do the current activity, and/or be prepared to introduce another. Always keep a close eye on the group, not just to show them that you think what they are doing is important, but also to enable you to be ready to change gears. During this activity, we quietly got together, confirmed our next step and went back to watching the group. When we presented the new version, the group had no idea that we had not planned it to go that way from the beginning.

Variation

If the wood is too low or too unsteady for your group, try using a longer piece of wood and balancing it on the backs of the chairs or between two tables. Then just mark off the size of the building area with tape. Keep in mind that changing the length and width of the wood and the number of objects will change the level of difficulty.

Items Needed:

2 chairs
3-foot length of 2"x4" board
2, 3-foot pieces of rope
10 to 15 odd objects (frisbee, ball, water balloon, hairbrush, old sneaker, ruler, etc.)

Group Size: **2 or more**

Format: **Group**

LOST YOUR MARBLES

Lost Your Marbles probably taxes frustration tolerance more than any other skill. Communication and coordination are also very important. Your debrief should touch on all of these areas.

Procedure

Round up about 50 marbles. Scatter them around the table. Be sure to first tape your empty gift wrap rolls (see items needed) around the edges of the table as bumpers or the marbles will soon be on the floor. Each person is seated next to his partner. Their inside arms (the arms that are closest to their partner) are loosely tied together with a blindfold at the wrist. For safety's sake, clients should be able to easily pull their arm out if they need to. Each person is given a plastic spoon to hold in his tethered hand. Each person in the pair must get a marble on their spoon before they can attempt to put them in their container. Give them about 10 minutes and then count up the marbles. The pair with the most wins. If your table is slanted and all the marbles roll to one side, or just for the fun of it, keep rolling the marbles around the table.

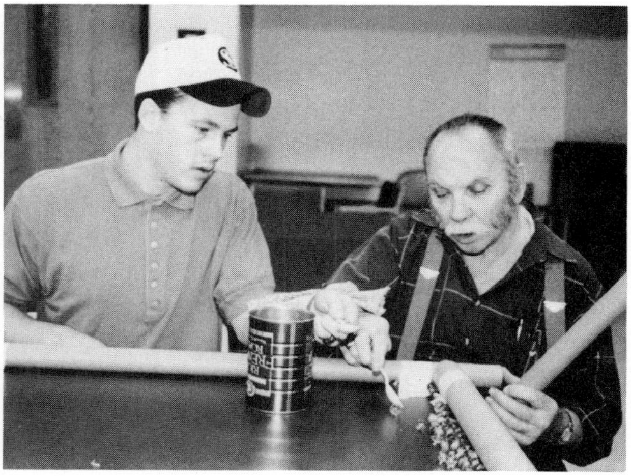

Next, have them use plastic knives. This time they need to work together and pick up one marble between them. This way is much more difficult. Other tools to try are chopsticks, emery boards and toilet paper rolls. Also, think about varying the openings of the containers, using anything from coffee cans to soda bottles.

You can take the emphasis off of competition in a couple of ways if it is likely to be an issue. You can set a goal that you think all of them can beat, say, five marbles. This number, though, is likely to change given what tools they're using and the opening size of their container. Then your quick tally in between rounds can be very positive: "Everyone has more than five marbles. You beat the World Record!" You have to be careful, though, and make sure everyone will beat it. The groups can predict what the next goal should be based on past performance and changes made. You can also have them switch partners so it is never the same team winning or losing. This change also reemphasizes communication every round as they have to figure out an approach with this new person.

Caution

Be aware that someone who has left-sided hemiplegia or ataxia will need to sit on the left side of the pair so his right arm is tied to the person next to him. Of course, he'll need to sit on the right side if he has right-sided deficits. We mention this issue so that you think about it beforehand and think about your clients' level of adjustment. You can easily plan seating and partner-changing in such a way that the person is on the correct side without any discussion. On the other hand, if the person needs to start dealing with recognizing and discussing his limits, you might have him sit on the "wrong" side of his partner and force a discussion between the two about his needs. This can be an especially normalizing or powerful discussion if both people are hemiplegic. The nice thing about *Lost Your Marbles* is that as long as the other arm and hand are unaffected, this team should not be at a disadvantage.

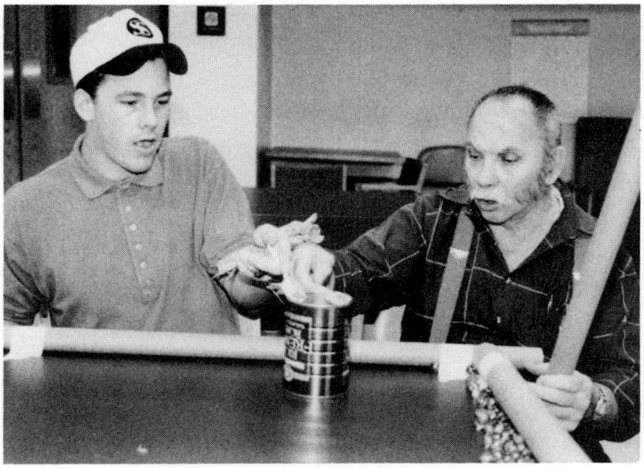

Debriefing

During the debrief you might encourage them to talk about the (lack of) role of the hemiplegia and brainstorm other daily activities that would be unaffected by the deficit. This discussion could then extend to activities that would be different but still possible. We're focused on hemiplegia, but you could really have this type of discussion with any number of activities and a variety of different deficits.

Items Needed:

50 marbles
1 jar or bottle or other container per pair
1 blindfold per pair (used as an arm tie)
1 plastic knife and spoon per person
empty gift wrap or paper towel rolls to be used as bumpers
tape

Group Size: **4 or more**

Format: **Pairs**

MOVE IT OR LOSE IT

The inspiration for *Move it or Lose it* came about when one of us (who shall remain nameless) needed to clean her house in a hurry, which is becoming quite a habit — speaking of planning deficits. So there she was, running frantically from one room to another downstairs, grabbing all the junk around that needed to go upstairs (into the back of a closet out of sight for the moment). Refusing to make two trips, she kept grabbing more and more. By the time she made it up to the closet, there was a trail of dropped stuff following her all the way up the steps. This story does have a happy ending, though. The company came and the house looked fine — no one checked the closets. Eventually the junk found its way out of the closet and rescattered itself around the house as all really good junk does. And we gained a fun group activity.

Procedure

In *Move it or Lose it,* the group must move a pile of objects from one designated place to another about twenty feet away in one trip without dropping anything. Of course, we have included rules to add to the excitement and challenge. Use the sample guide sheet on the next page or create your own. Notice rule #6. This rule stops members from working in isolation. Predicting the number of rule violations (at the bottom of the guide sheet) helps the group to remember to stop and consult the rules and to act less on impulse. Rules 7 and 8 are the ones to keep your eyes on: each person may use only one hand at a time and no one may put anything on themself to transport. Inevitably, the group gets to the last item, someone picks it up and off they go. No good. Sound the buzzer. It is also not acceptable for someone else to put down one of their items, hand the last item to someone and then pick their old item back up. Although it may not sound that difficult, we had a couple of groups get to this point and run out of time as they debated what to do.

Everyone may be given a guide sheet so that everyone is accountable, but we also ask for a volunteer to serve as a Rule Monitor. Having a piece of paper to refer to also helps to compensate for memory deficits. Or, if you prefer, read the rules out loud and have the group take notes.

Use the Items Needed list below as a guide. Add, subtract or modify anything on the list. As always, use whatever you can most easily gather.

In addition to communication, this activity targets planning. House cleaning is an optional debriefing topic.

Items Needed:

water balloon
hula hoop
balls
basket
hat
gloves
apron
plant
ice
life jacket
etc...
piece of paper
racquet
long piece of wood
pencil
scarf
vest
egg
ball with soap on it
container of water (no lid)
umbrella

Group Size: **3 or more**

Format: **Group**

MOVE IT OR LOSE IT

Guide Sheet

Object: To move all of the objects from Point A to Point B without dropping anything.

Rules:

1) Make one trip only as a group.
2) If anything is dropped, the entire group must go back and start again.
3) Everyone must transport something.
4) If clothing is worn, only 2 pieces may be worn by each person.
5) The piece of paper must be returned as is (no wrinkles, folds, etc.).
6) When moving from A to B, the group must be connected or touching in some way; i.e., you must move as a whole.
7) Everyone may use only one hand at any time.
8) No one may put anything on themselves to transport, but you may help others to load up with their cargo.

Predicted Number of Rule Violations:

Rule Monitor:

MYSTERY CLUE HUNT

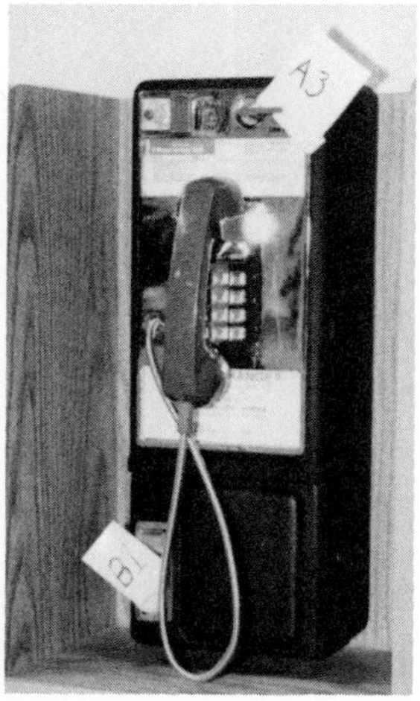

Clue Hunts require some planning, but they are well worth the effort because of the enthusiasm they create in groups of all ages. This version is filled with mystery, suspense and competition. Before the group gathers, the leaders must create clues that will lead the teams from one chosen place to the next. They must then place each clue and a prop in a specific location. For example, the first clue handed to the group might read, "Don't call me, I'll call you," leading them to another clue taped to the side of a phone. There they will also find a prop — maybe sunglasses. The clue on the phone might say, "I can't believe I ate the whole thing." The group puts their heads together and decides to check out the lunch room. There they find another clue and a beach ball. The theme is beginning to unravel. Then on to the next clue. It's enlightening for the therapists to quietly follow along and watch the group's problem-solving skills at work.

Procedure

At the beginning of the session, divide the group into two teams, which compete against each other, to be the first to unravel the theme of the hunt. (Notice that you will need two sets of props and two sets of clues.) Start the activity with the group leader saying, "In a few minutes you will be handed a clue to solve. This clue will lead you to another where you will also find a prop. Follow all of the clues and collect all of your team's props. Put all of your props together at the end and try to solve your team's theme."

You will need to tailor your clues to refer to specific places within your own building or department. You may use as many clues as you think time will allow, given the difficulty of the clues, the distances they will need to travel, and the level of your group.

Within our forty-five minute sessions, we find that five clues work best for the level of our clients. Remember that while one team is heading off in one direction, the other team will be heading off in another, so two therapists will be needed. Although, if you have a small group, you could have them work together in one group.

During processing, we often need to discuss impulsivity, teamwork and sharing ideas. We frequently have one or two members who will get an idea and then run off to pursue it, leaving the others behind. The responsibility for making sure everyone is involved should, however, lie with everyone. So if someone reported that his teammates didn't share their ideas, you might question what he could have done. He could have asked the others what was going on. Below are some rules to read to the group before sending them off. Rule #1 fosters time management, and Rule #2 encourages group communication.

Rules: (As always, subject to change.)

1) You must return to the room by ____ (5–7 minutes before the group officially ends) — even if your group is not done.
2) Include every member of the team in on problem solving whenever possible.

Possible themes and props include:

- Beach Party — sunglasses, sun block, towel, plastic bucket, Bermuda shorts, etc.
- Mystery — trench coat, pipe, fingerprint, magnifying glass, small note pad, etc.
- Holiday — items chosen to reflect an upcoming holiday
- Occupation — any job can be chosen (ex.: teacher - apple, chalk, pointer, red pen, stickers, ruler)
- Birthday Party — candles, streamers, gift wrapped box, party favors, donkey tails

Items Needed: **clues**
props — see lists above

Group Size: **4 or more**

Format: **Group vs. Group**
Pairs
Group

THE NAME GAME

Anyone who recognizes *The Name Game* has probably spent too much time at parties with their friends. *The Name Game* is excellent for addressing speed of processing, divergent thinking and word finding. It is best used when your primary activity ends early and you have some time left. If we have the opportunity, we'll do it more than once with the same group so we can see if they remember it and can use strategies learned previously.

Procedure

With everyone sitting in a circle, one person begins by saying the name of someone famous. The name could be of someone in the movies, on television, in the news, in politics, a famous criminal, an athlete ...anyone recognizable. If someone has never heard the name and challenges, it must be corroborated by at least two other people. If two other people have not heard the name it cannot be used and the next person starts off with a new name.

Hint: *Read this next sentence slowly*! Once someone has given a name, the person to their left must say another name *whose first name begins with the first letter of the previous name's last name.* It's actually not as confusing as it sounds. Here's an example. If the first person says Charlie Brown, the next person may say Billie Jean King because Billie begins with the same letter as Charlie's *last* name. After Billie Jean King, you might hear Kathleen Turner and then Ted Turner, Tammy Wynette, Willie Nelson, and so on. Got it? Notice that the same rule applies even if the first and last names begin with the same letter.

Even though the pressure is on each individual for coming up with a name when it is his turn, there are no consequences and it is guaranteed that almost everyone will be at a loss for a name at one time or another. You can give hints to someone if they are really stuck or you can make things harder by imposing a time limit for saying each new name. The leaders should participate in *The Name Game* so that the clients can see what "normal" speed of processing would be like. (That last statement assumes a lot about the abilities of the group leaders!)

Debriefing

During our debriefing sessions, we talk a lot about speed of processing since decreased speed of processing and head injury seem to go hand in hand. Often we will stop *The Name Game* part way through so that we can discuss the issue and then some strategies while there's still an opportunity to try them out. A strategy to increase speed and word retrieval in this activity might be to think of any first name that begins with the letter you need and then try to match a famous last name to that. It usually helps. After the discussion, continue on and see if the strategy use improves performance. At the end, you can contrast the performance before and after the strategy was discussed, then talk about other situations where speed is important and what they might do.

Group Size: **3 or more**

Format: **Group**

NO SNEEZING!

The object of *No Sneezing* is simple — build! The bigger, the better. Remember building card houses as a kid? That's what *No Sneezing* is all about. Standard playing cards are fine, but we prefer pieces of cardboard. We cut up the cardboard backs of writing tablets (we never throw anything out!) into four fairly equal pieces. They are sturdier and easier to handle than playing cards, but only slightly less frustrating. Although now that we think about it, it would be fun to try using full size pieces of cardboard! Hmm ...next time. Hand the group a pile of pieces and let them go. The only rule, as always, is that everyone must be involved. Oh, and ...no sneezing!

Processing issues might include coordination, communication, creativity, planning and, don't forget, frustration tolerance.

Variations:

- Play team versus team.
- Play group versus leaders (you know you'd love to try it!).
- Use playing cards.
- Use Legos or Tinkertoys — easier, but they allow more room for creativity.
- Use greeting cards or note cards — easier to build with than cardboard because of the fold.
- Use file folders and build on the floor.
- Follow a diagram.
- Create a diagram from their own building before it falls down.
- Follow written directions.
- Assign Builders and Architects — Architects give directions and answer questions, but can't touch. Then switch roles.

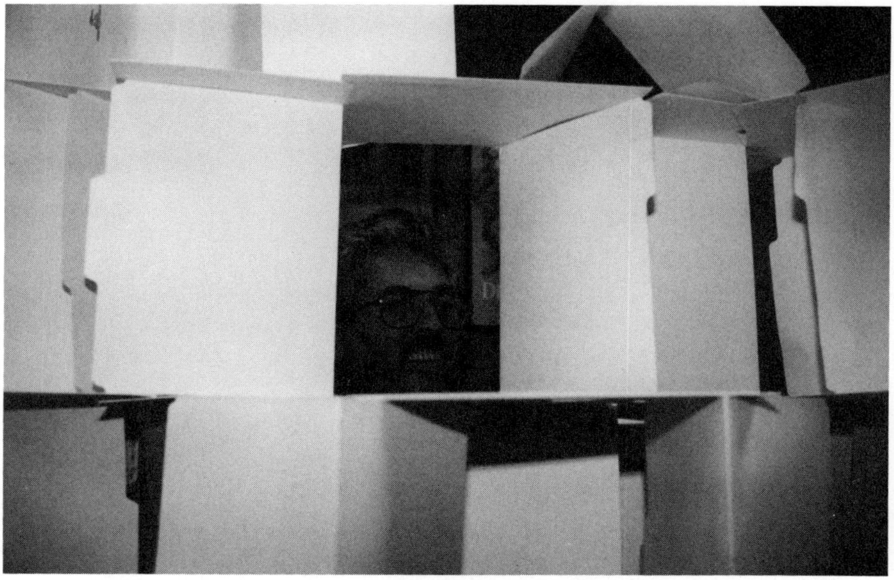

- Use one hand.
- Build according to categories — tallest, skinniest, fattest, most unique, etc.
- Build specified buildings — a town hall, a mansion, the Eiffel Tower, the Empire State Building, a firehouse.
- Add other props in — toothpicks, pencils, post-it paper.
- Use tape if the group lacks the fine motor control necessary.

Items Needed: **standard playing cards**
cardboard squares
greeting cards or manila folders
Other items may be required depending on the variation chosen above.

Group Size: **2 or more**

Format: **Group**
Group vs. Group
Pairs

ONE LUMP OR TWO?

One Lump or Two helps you turn a vice into a fun activity. Save the cans accumulated from your morning coffee. Punch four holes around the bottom edges of several coffee cans and run two pieces of string through two holes each. Give a can to each person in the group. The object is for them to pass a ball (golf, tennis, beach) from person to person via the coffee cans attached to various parts of their bodies.

Procedure

You can have them pass in a variety of ways. They may each be given the same body part to tie the can to like their head, shoulder or stomach. Or you can have them choose. You can even specify that no two people may have it tied to the same place. Hands may not be used to steady the cans. You can increase memory demands by having the ball passed around several times, without being passed in the same order twice. They can pass several balls in their cans at the same time (as long as you are using small enough ones). Or as soon as one ball is passed start another. With this last one, it is fun to impose a holding time limit. For instance, you may not hold onto a ball for more than ten seconds. This means that if the person directly next to you is not yet ready to receive a ball, you had better quickly find someone else who is!

Have fun and keep them moving.

When you're done, discuss good places to have had the coffee cans versus bad ones, communication, coordination, speed, and memory.

Items Needed: 1 coffee can for each person
string
tennis, golf or beach balls

Group Size: 5 or more

Format: Group

ORB ESCAPE

While looking for intelligent life, an alien orb becomes trapped underground in an Earthly sewer system. The orb must escape quickly because his spaceship is about to take off and return home. The group must choose to work together to help the orb escape. The orb is actually a marble, superball or other type of small ball. The escape route is an underground pipeline (empty cardboard gift wrap rolls). Each person is given a piece of "pipe" which they can only hold with one hand. The orb must pass through all of the hand held pipes without falling out in order to escape.

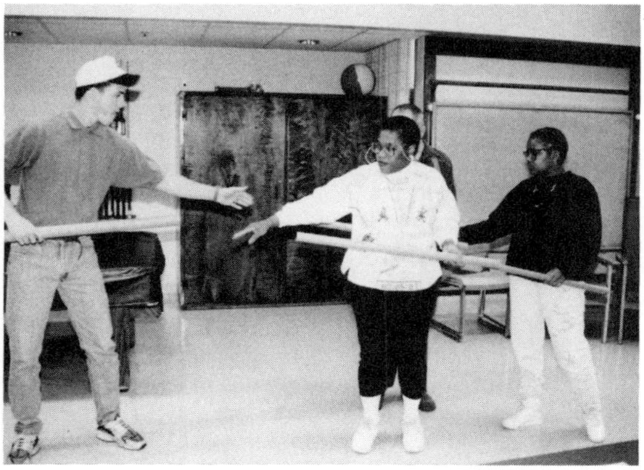

Procedure

The group stands in a line, holding their rolls end to end and the marble, or rather, the orb is placed in the first one and rolls all the way through to the end. Depending on the group and the way they choose to solve this challenge, it may not be too difficult for them. So, give them some new challenges:

1) Put more than one orb in the escape route at a time (you may want to put a basket or bucket at the end to catch the flying orbs!).
2) The orb must travel very fast (time them and then see if they can beat that time).
3) The orb must travel very slowly (this is tough — again, time them and have them try again).

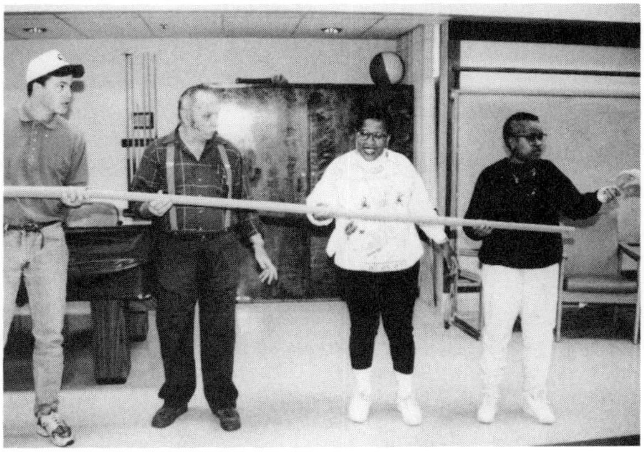

4) Stop the orb before it comes out the end (without touching it) and send it back the other way.
5) Pass the orb in a continuous circle.
6) Make the orb bounce on the floor once before being caught by the next person in their pipe.
7) Leaders — join in for extra bodies.
8) Everyone gets a paper towel roll in each hand. You may not pass to yourself. Try all of the above in this new formation.

Items Needed: **marbles or other small balls**
various sized paper rolls like from gift wrap or paper towels

Group Size: **4 or more**

Format: **Group**

PACK YOUR BAGS

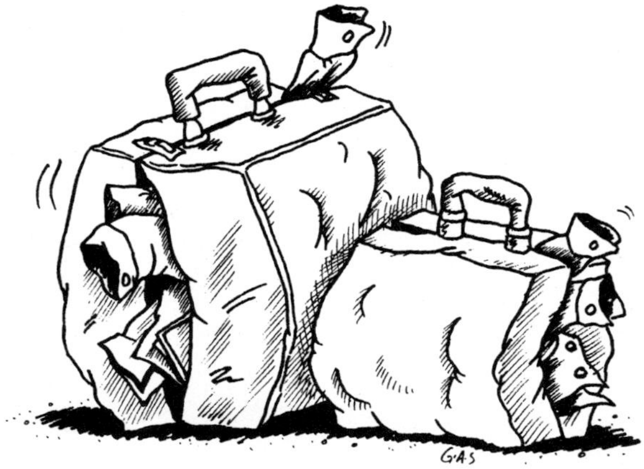

Pack Your Bags is a good follow-up activity to *Pile-on.* Since the skills involved, especially planning, are very similar, it provides you with an opportunity to see if the group can generalize their skills to a new situation. You can have them do *Pack Your Bags* during the next session or wait awhile.

Procedure

For *Pack Your Bags,* you will need a medium-sized suitcase, preferably with several outside pockets, and lots of other "stuff." See the list below for some suggestions. Throw the pile of stuff and the suitcase on the table. Tell the group that you are going on a trip to see your sister in California. Of course, if you live in California you'll have to pick some other far away exotic place — like New Jersey! Tell the group that you need their help packing. They need to write up a plan of how the suitcase should be packed, but they should not actually pack anything. You will need to be able to understand and follow their plan when you pack your bag tomorrow.

There are a few things that we definitely like to try to include each time. In the pile of stuff is usually a small box and a beautiful pair of plastic earrings. This is a gift for your sister. To go along with it is a roll of wrapping paper that is too big to fit inside the suitcase. If they decide to cut the paper and/or wrap the present and leave the roll behind, that is fine. We also have a bottle of shampoo that has been entirely slimed with the shampoo or dish detergent or something. There is always a plastic bag in the pile, too. Act surprised when they find out that the bottle is slimed and tell them how very important it is that your clothes do not get slimed up in the suitcase because you will need to wear them to a surprise birthday party. It would be nice if these party clothes could be pants with paint on them and an oversized flannel shirt. ("I do like to look my best!") Once we even included a cupcake (for the birthday!) and a Tupperware container. There should be enough items so that the planning is actually a challenge, but not so many that they would not be able to get everything in.

When they are done and you are able to understand their plan (thank them profusely), you can have them pack the bag or you can do it so that they can see their plan in action.

Debriefing

Their actual packing success or failure provides content for debriefing. You'll want to talk about how they planned, how they communicated, and the clarity of their written plan. You might also discuss what they might change when they help you pack your bags for that trip you've always wanted to take to Colorado. How do you get skis into a suitcase anyway?

Items Needed:

roll of gift wrap
plastic earrings or the like
painter's pants
boots
book
cassettes
plastic bag
cupcake
brush
soap
sweater, etc.
small box
flannel shirt
gardening gloves
socks
writing pad
shampoo (slimed)
rubber band
Tupperware
old battered toothbrush
belt

Group Size: **2 or more**

Format: **Group**

PASSING LANE

Passing Lane requires hand-holding and standing close together. Be sure your group can deal with that, especially if you're working with adolescents. You don't need a lot of room. We usually use a lightly traveled hallway.

Procedure

To create a *Passing Lane*, have the group divide in half and form two parallel lines facing each other. The more people the better in this one, so feel free to join in. The first thing the group has to do is reach across and join hands with two other people. As they are doing this, you should tell them that they should create as tight a *Passing Lane* as possible because they will have to — you guessed it — pass things along. Therefore, they will not want to have a lot of gaps between their arms. If they want to rearrange things, let them. Wheelchairs are no problem, the group will just have to adjust themselves to accommodate the variations in arm height. Let them figure out how.

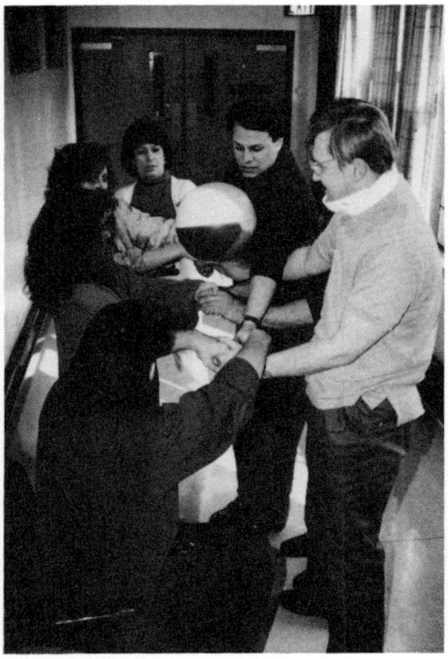

Before beginning, warn clients of any range of motion limitations. Just to be sure, you may want to ask if anyone will have any problems if their arms go over a specific height. Remember that two other people will be holding onto their arms so they will not be in complete control of their own arms. If you have a question about the group's ability to remember the limits or control their behavior in the moment, you can position yourself so that you are holding the hand of the person with the restricted range of motion.

When they are ready, start big and easy by passing a beach ball down the lane. Let them try it a few times so they get good at it and begin to feel comfortable. Don't be surprised if the ball goes flying outside the *Passing Lane* over their heads once in a while. This is part of the fun. Then switch to a volleyball, tennis ball and eventually a golf ball, letting them try each one a couple of times. You can give each new ball a big build-up and ask them to predict how well they'll do with each new challenge.

Have them switch places periodically so that they need to work with different people. There is no reason not to try to pass some unorthodox things, like blindfolds, balloons, Tupperware and rope! During the debrief, encourage the group to discuss the differences between the objects and any effects they may have had on their problem-solving and communication.

Items Needed:

beach ball
volleyball
tennis ball
golf ball
blindfold (optional)
Tupperware (optional)
rope (optional)
balloon (optional)

Group Size: **6 or more**

Format: **Group**

PILE-ON

You be the judge on this one. We've designed this activity to rely heavily on planning skills. These crucial skills are often difficult ones for many populations. Emphasize teamwork and sharing ideas in addition to planning. *Pile-On* is harder that you initially might think.

Procedure

Gather 20 to 25 varied objects and lay them out on the table. In the center of the table, set out a board (approximately 2 feet by 1 foot) which has about a 9 by 12 inch area marked off in the center. This area is the only space which can be built on. The therapists are "county officials" in *Pile-On*. Start by telling the group that they are architects who need to create a building (otherwise known as a *Pile-On* structure). Then read to them the county codes below. The directions and county codes may only be discussed with the county officials for the first five minutes, so encourage note taking. When the five minutes are up, sit back and watch the action unfold....

Their structure must incorporate all of the objects supplied. But before building, they must submit a written plan and/or diagram to the county officials to see if it meets the county building codes. The plan must be extremely clear. The county officials should not need to make any assumptions about where anything is going to be placed. The county officials will review the plan and note any violation, for example, extending the foundation beyond the designated boundaries. If it is turned down, they will be told why and given an opportunity to modify the plan. After the plan has been accepted, the group must then use their plan to construct their *Pile-On* structure. Watch out for the water balloon!! If their plan does not work, it's back to the drawing board!

We once had a group whose plan we knew was not very clear. We had made several comments questioning it, but they assured us that it was perfectly fine. We knew that they knew where they wanted everything to be placed. So, to have them build based on their plan would not show them where the problems were. In fact, because they had gone over it so many times, they probably didn't even need to follow their plan at all. Our next thought was for us to use their plan and build the structure. But that had it's downside too. We had been watching them for the past couple of sessions while they planned, so we knew where they intended everything to go as well. Also, if we messed something up and told them it was unclear, they would have probably blamed it on us and not the plan. We probably would have, too. We were clearly biased at that point. But still, they needed the feedback. What to do?

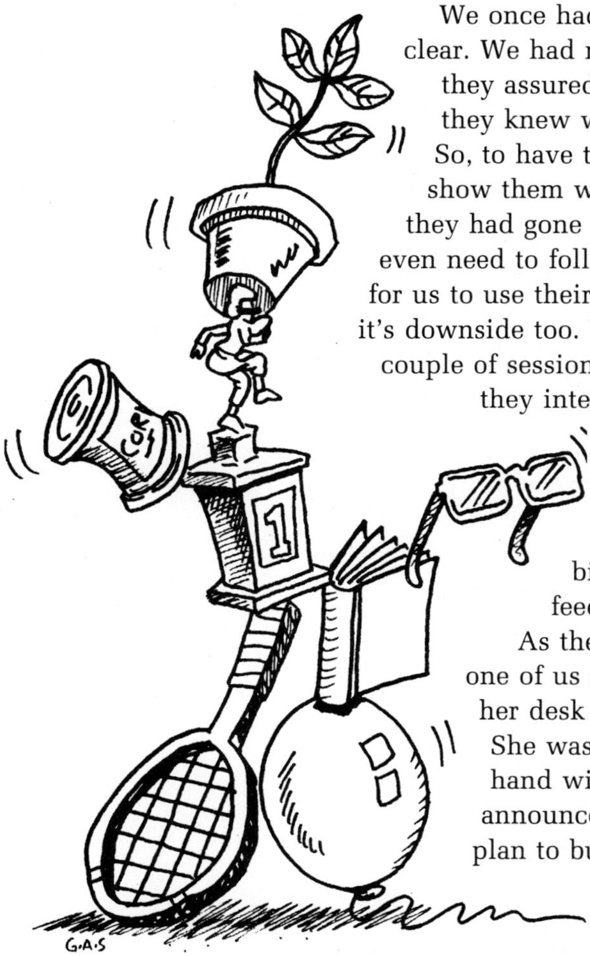

As they were going over their plan one last time, one of us slipped out into the staff office. Sitting at her desk was an unsuspecting speech pathologist. She was quickly led back to the group to "give us a hand with something". Before she could object, we announced that Eileen here was going to use their plan to build their *Pile-On*. Well, she made almost every wrong move we had anticipated and a couple of others. The group had some great visual feedback and validated every bit of it. We highly recommend this approach. We're likely to use it most of the time again in the future. Probably the only time we wouldn't use it would be if we felt it was more important that the group experience success. Then we would allow them to build.

Pile-On is very challenging. Another group spent two sessions trying to come up with a plan. They became very frustrated and swore it could not be done. Their communication, planning and organization were poor and they could not find a way to make it successful. So, on the third day, the group leaders solved it, modeling ways of structuring, planning, asking questions and explaining to each other reasons behind ideas. On the same day they watched a video of their performance and compared the approaches. This mix of experiential learning and modeling enabled them to figure out where they could improve. Two weeks later, the group made another *Pile-On* attempt (using different objects and codes, of course), and their planning and communication were more successful.

You can use the county codes listed below or make up your own based on the objects you have available. The codes add to the need for note taking and require managing multiple pieces of information. They can be added to or even totally eliminated, depending on the cognitive skills of your group.

COUNTY BUILDING CODES

1) You must use the board provided as your foundation. Nothing may touch the board outside the designated area, however, objects can hang over it.
2) All items given must be included on the *Pile-On*.
3) You must submit a plan to the county officials for approval before building. During this planning stage you may work with a maximum of two things at a time to see if your design idea will work. Before trying a new idea, you must disassemble the first two. For example, you may see if the ball fits inside the cup, but then you must disassemble them before trying to see if the fan will stand up in the skein of yarn.
4) The fan must be opened when on the *Pile-On* structure.
5) The lollipop must stand on one of its ends.
6) The pine cone may not be placed inside anything.

Items Needed:

1 board approximately 2 feet by 1 foot
water balloon
hanger
bottle of hand cream
wash cloth
drinking glass
small ball
Christmas ornament
plastic spoon
paper plate
pine cone
skein of yarn
fan
magazine
can of tennis balls
box of cereal
lei
sunglasses
dowel

Group Size: **2 or more**

Format: **Group**

PILE-ON COMPETITION

This *Pile-On* variation involves group versus group competition. Our groups have always dealt with competition in a positive way. They focus on what and how their team has done rather than whether they won or lost. Keep in mind, and help them keep in mind, that it's possible to win but do a poor job along the way. Take out the competitive aspect if you need to and keep the debrief focused on the process and not on the win or loss.

Procedure

A barrier (cardboard, bulletin board, etc.) is placed between the two groups. They are each given a pile of similar objects. They must build their *Pile-On* structure according to your description. Some examples are the highest, the smallest base, or the most original. Or you can tell them that it must look like something when it is done (other than a building, of course). They decide what that "something" will be. One point is awarded to the team that builds theirs the fastest, in order to encourage efficiency. Two points are awarded to the team that wins in the particular category; i.e., whoever actually has the highest structure, or smallest base, etc.. When possible, have the individuals decide who won. If they are competitive, they may continually vote for themselves, though, and you'll have a perpetual tie!

Unlike the first *Pile-On* version, we do not make them plan these structures out ahead of time, but you could if it better suited your goals. Here our emphasis is more on group cooperation and communication. We also do not always give them county codes to use. Keep this variation in mind in case the first one ends too soon and you need to take up some time.

Items Needed: large barrier
2 sets of about 20 identical or very similar objects — see Pile-On for ideas

Group Size: 4 or more

Format: Group vs. Group
Group
Pairs

THE PIT

Don't be scared away by the list of equipment for *The Pit*. You can use any pile of stuff that you have available. Go to your cabinet or box or co-workers' desks and just start gathering. The only things that are necessary as these instructions are written are the dowels, or similar items, like tennis racquets.

Procedure

In the center of a big room, or outside, make a large circle with rope, string, tape or chalk. Put a bunch of objects in the circle, scattered all about. The group is divided into teams or pairs. Each person is given a 3-foot dowel or something similar. Each team (or pair) must use the dowels to lift and carry — not slide — as many objects from *The Pit* as possible. Some of the objects may be difficult to reach or awkward to grab (especially by a single person with a single dowel), ...that's what they must work out, problem solve and communicate together!

Initially, clients may only use the dowels to retrieve the objects, but once they get a nice collection, they can use those objects to assist in the retrieval of the ones that might still be stuck in the middle of *The Pit* or be more awkward to grab. Watch out, though. If whatever they decide to use falls back into *The Pit,* they must get it back out again in order to get points for it. While it is in the middle, it becomes fair game and is at risk for being snatched up by the competition. To add more excitement, we tell the group that they are allowed to interfere with what the other team is doing. They may use their dowels to push away an object that the other team is trying to retrieve from *The Pit*. This encourages them to be concerned not only with what their own team is doing, but also with what the other team is up to. If you have very nice, polite teams, you may want to involve yourself in this activity and make the first move toward disrupting the other team. Believe us, the other team *will* retaliate! When time is up, see who has the most objects and then process the experience. Depending on how things went, frustration tolerance might be a good subject to talk about.

To defuse an intensely competitive situation (or to add a little twist just for fun), holler "switch partners" or "switch teams" at key points in the middle of play. They must immediately stop what they are doing and change. We learned firsthand what this felt like during a PA workshop. It makes great material for processing, especially when someone who was playing all-out now finds himself on the team that is behind!

Items needed:

rope, string, tape or chalk (to make the pit)
1 three foot dowel (or similar object) for each person
tennis ball
pen
doll
block
sneaker
hat
tissue
rock
book
shaving cream on a piece of plastic wrap??
feather
magazine
deck of cards
shampoo bottle
nail polish
stapler
etc.

Group Size: **4 or more**

Format:

Group vs. Group
Pairs

ROAD TRIP

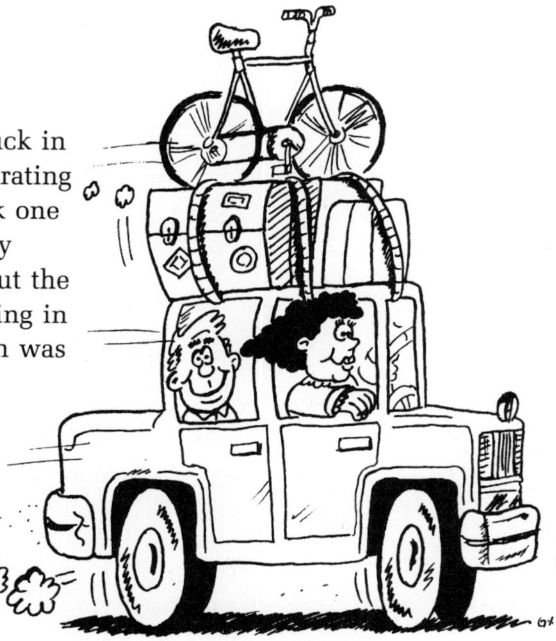

If you've ever been stuck in traffic, you know how frustrating it can be. I was put to work one day after complaining to my Initiative Group buddy about the amount of traffic I was hitting in the morning. Her suggestion was to look for unique license plates — the ones that say something. She thought we could collect a bunch of them and use them in an activity. So that's what I did and then even thought up some of my own. Well, it did help my commute a bit, at least for awhile, *and* we got a challenging activity out of it. Thanks, Wendy! So, here they are! You can use our license plates and add some of your own.

Procedure

Put each license plate on a 3"x5" index card. You can use them for the whole group or make a second set and divide the group into two competing teams. Give them a time limit and see who can solve the most. If needed, a simple way to make them easier is to put a space break where each word or syllable would end. After they have tried a few, help them to discuss the strategies they are using in order to solve the license plates. Then help them, as needed, to apply these strategies to the more difficult ones. We have found ourselves becoming more active in *Road Trip* than in some of the other activities because of the cognitive flexibility and problem-solving required. Discuss the need for these skills during the brief and debrief.

Here are some of those strategies we mentioned. To be fair, don't read these until you have tried solving the license plates.

1) Sometimes a letter makes its sound — the letter k = "kuh"
2) Sometimes a letter says its name — the letter k = "kay"
3) Sometimes letters or numbers stand alone.
4) Sometimes letters or numbers are grouped with the others next to them.
5) Sometimes the only problem is that the vowels are missing.

Try to solve the license plates yourself before you look at the answers! Some are extremely difficult.

Variation

Hold up the license plate on a flash card for about 10–15 seconds and then take it away in order to increase attention, memory and/or note taking.

LICENSE PLATES:	**ANSWERS:**
OPR2NIT	Opportunity
PLABAL	Playball
KRMT	Kermit
EZDSIT	Easy Does It
SWTSTF	Sweet Stuff
NGINEAR	Engineer
RKTEKT	Architect
4U2C	For You To See
GRMTCHF	Gourmet Chef
10SNE1	Tennis Anyone
XTC	Ecstacy
MKYMSE	Mickey Mouse
ATOPLT	Auto Pilot
ILVMNY	I Love Money
ILVDGS	I Love Dogs
WKGWMN	Working Woman
XLNT	Excellent
4FDGRPS	Four Food Groups

LICENSE PLATES:	ANSWERS:
BALUCNB	Be All You Can Be
CULTR	See You Later
WHTSNU	What's New
URNDIT	Earned It
BUTFL	Beautiful
FSTLNE	Fast Lane
25 BACK	Quarterback
GDGRF	Good Grief
GMSTMTCH	Game, Set, Match
IIII	Four Eyes
LVNITUP	Living It Up
22	Tu-tu
LAFINT	Elephant
DUXOUP (Bonus Points!)	Duck Soup

Items Needed: **license plates written on index cards or a blackboard and chalk**

Group Size: **3 or more**

Format: **Group**
Group vs. Group

ROCKY ROAD

Remember as a kid crossing a creek by jumping from one slippery, shaky rock to another? Well, that is what *Rocky Road* is all about except that, in true Initiative Group style, there are some rules. The object is for the entire group to get from one side of the "creek" to the other. Each person may only step on rocks that are designated as theirs either by color, number, letter, etc. (see exception below). These rocks can be anything that won't slide and big enough to step on with both feet.

Procedure

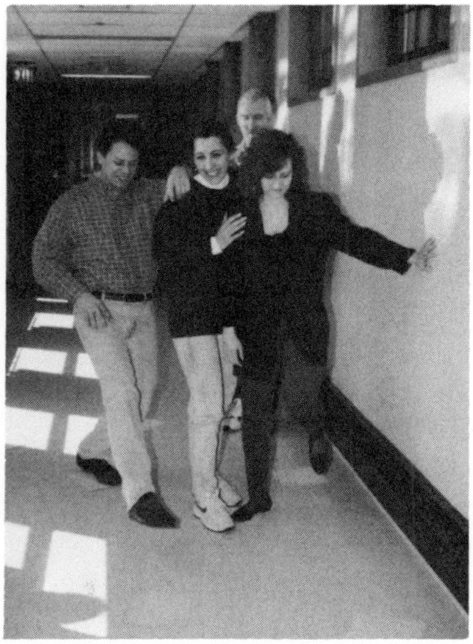

The rocks are scattered about on the floor so that it would be a challenge for someone to make it across without support from others or without needing to step on someone else's rock. The layout below works well for five people and can easily be adjusted to work for more or less people. Leaders can join in, but should not be active problem solvers.

Another person's rock can only be stepped on if the "owner" is on the rock at the same time. You can make a couple of big rocks and arrange the layout in such a way that they will be likely to need three people on a rock at the same time. No one may step backward at any time, nor can they step off of a rock. If they realize that it is not possible to go any further given the choices they have made, the group should go back to the beginning and try again. Encourage them to think it through and plan before they begin so that they rely more on problem-solving and less on trial and error. You can approach this additional attempt as another chance to succeed using what they learned the first time rather than as a failure.

Since there are several rules, we hand out a rule sheet (see the example). We read through the rules with them and physically demonstrate each one. After an initial period for asking questions is over, we refer them back to the rule sheet and each other for further clarification.

Make rules regarding jumping as they make sense for your group. If they can handle it physically, then allow them to, but only if you are confident your rocks won't slide. As in other activities, do not worry about wheelchairs, canes, or walkers touching forbidden territory (in this case, the water). Just worry about feet.

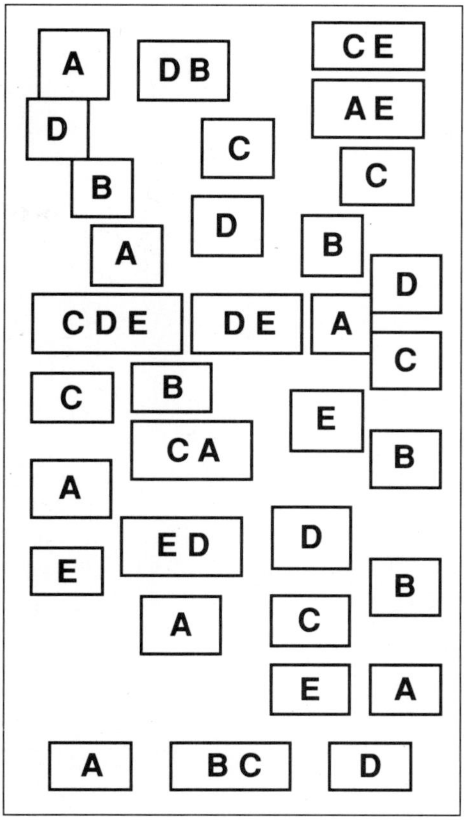

Debriefing

Processing topics include: comparing one attempt versus another, problem-solving approach, communication, need for reliance on others (sharing rocks), learning (the complex directions) and memory (for rules and directions).

Items Needed: **several rubber mats or pieces of paper to serve as rocks**

Group Size: **3 or more**

Format: **Group**

ROCKY ROAD RULE SHEET

Object: **To get the entire group to the other side.**

1) You must step primarily on the rocks that *you* own. You do not need to step on all of your rocks.
2) You may not step backwards.
3) You may step on a rock that belongs to another person if and only if the owner is on the rock at the same time. The owner may not leave until you leave.
4) You may not share a rock with the same person two times in a row.
5) No jumping. Instead, if you need help moving from one rock to another, ask for help from your group.
6) If you get to a point where you realize that one or all of you cannot make it the entire way, everyone must go back to the beginning and try a new approach.

SACRED CHALICE RESCUE

Sacred Chalice Rescue is always well received by our groups. As with all of the activities, you can choose the story we have here in order to add a little drama and excitement, or you can eliminate it and give them the rules and guidelines in a straight forward manner. Which you choose to do will depend on the makeup of your group. Think of this as a mile relay event in the Olympics, where the baton is passed from one runner to the next. Only here, there are restrictions on how to pass and carry the baton (or sacred chalice).

Procedure

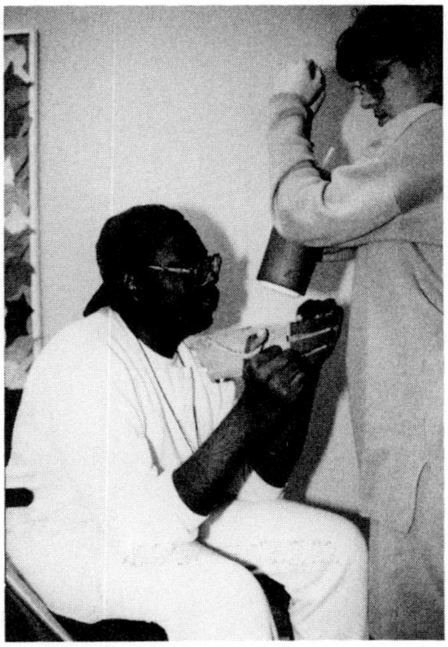

The therapist should tell the group: "You are all secret agents from different countries with different customs and ways of operating. You have been chosen to represent your country because of your special talents. Your mission is to get the sacred chalice (any cup will do!) from enemy territory to safety by working cooperatively with all the other agents. But, you must observe each agent's special way of operating and adhere to the international laws."

The therapists should pick any two fairly close points to be their start and end points. For example, they might go from one end of a hallway to the other. Make the points far enough apart, though, so that they may not simply pass the chalice from one to the other but will need to travel. In this way, they will need to incorporate all of the customs suggested below. For instance, Turkey and Russia's customs involve travel. If the start and end points are too close together, these customs can be ignored. Each person is given an envelope containing the rule he or she must follow. Let the group figure out that they need to share their customs with everyone else. They are then responsible for making sure that everyone obeys their customs the international laws.

Most of the time we've done *Sacred Chalice Rescue,* we've had one or two people kind of hang back, especially in the beginning. The others are so involved in getting things going that they don't realize they've left someone out. One of us hangs back with them and says, "I don't know what's going on right now, do you?" This comment does two things. It gives them a subtle cue that they need to get in there and find out what's going on. It also plants a seed so that when we debrief and ask, "Did everyone always know what was happening?" — it may spark a memory. You can refer them back to international law #2, which says that everyone needs to be involved.

Possible International Laws

(read to the group)

1) Each agent must touch/carry the chalice twice and only twice. These two times may not be in a row.
2) The agents must all be involved in the decision making. Because the countries do not trust each other, a move cannot be made unless all agents know about it.

Possible Customs

(give one in an envelope to each group member)

a) Zimbabwe: You may carry the chalice only with your elbows.
b) Turkey: You may not move forward when you hold the chalice.
c) Canada: You may not accept the chalice from the agent from Turkey.
d) Russia: You may only move a total of two feet any time you hold the chalice.
e) Germany: You may not touch the chalice. You must use your country's sacred carrier (basket, paper bag, etc.).

Add to this list as needed in order to accommodate the size of your group.

Debriefing

The way the group went about solving the dilemma is a good topic for debriefing. We've seen *Sacred Chalice Rescue* done a few times in a very random fashion. They looked for who else was around who needed to go, without any thought about that agent's custom or the distance left to travel. Discuss the merits and/or problems of this approach. Often, the groups will not share their individual customs before beginning. Discuss where this lack of communication may have gotten in the way.

Items needed: **basket, cup, etc. to serve as the Sacred Chalice**
envelopes with customs in them — one for each person
paper bag or basket — to serve as Germany's sacred carrier

Group Size: **4 or more**

Format: **Group**

SCALE THE WALL

Scale the Wall is a fun, full body activity. At first glance it appears easy, but that is not necessarily so. It involves communication, coordination and thinking ahead. It is also a good activity for working on upper extremity range of motion goals.

Procedure

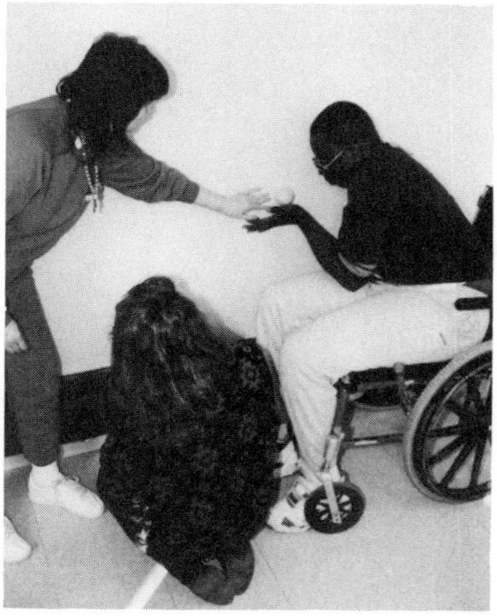

The object in *Scale the Wall* is for pairs to roll a ball from the floor up a wall to the ceiling (or a mark high on the wall) and back down using a prop. The people in the pairs must alternate after each turn. A turn is over when someone has rolled the ball up the wall the length of his prop. To get the idea, try this. Put a tennis ball on a wall, holding it there with your fingertips. Now start rolling it up the wall by moving it along your palm, then your forearm, then your upper arm. It will probably become out of reach or too awkward to manage just before it reaches your armpit. (See photos.) As another example, if I were using a tennis racquet as my prop, I would put the top of my racquet at the base of the ball. As I roll the ball up along my racquet, I will eventually get to the end of my racket. This marks the end of my turn and my partner must continue rolling from there with his own prop.

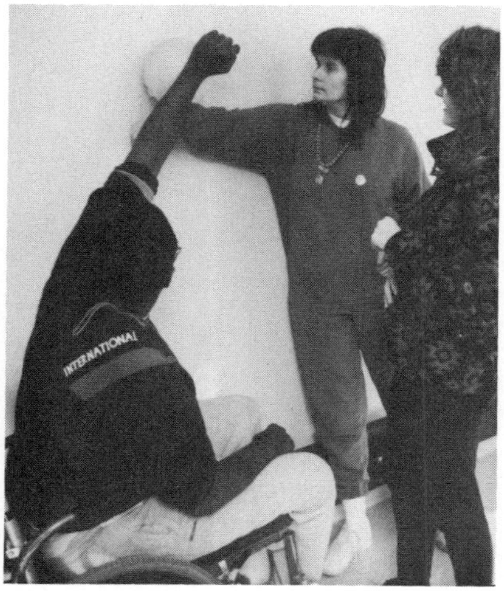

If the ball begins to fall, they need to try to catch it

by pressing it against the wall. They continue from wherever they catch it. If the ball hits the floor, they must start from the beginning.

Modifications:

There are lots of potential ways to play around with this seemingly easy activity.

- Vary the size of the props, so that they will move the ball for varying distances.
- Vary the number of people in the group; i.e., do not restrict it to pairs.
- Give the pairs a number of props, not allowing them to duplicate the use of one until all have been used once. Have one long prop to help them reach the ceiling. They will have to plan when to use each prop so that the long one is available to get the ball to the ceiling.
- Time them. Have the pairs play against the "world record" and not themselves.
- Holler, "switch!" and have the pairs change around.
- Switch props midway through.
- Have them do it several times, each time with a progressively smaller ball.
- Instead of using props, let clients use different parts of their bodies. They will have to get pretty close to each other, so make sure they are ready to handle it. This is actually our favorite way of having them *Scale the Wall.* We usually do not divide them into pairs. Instead, we let them figure out the best passing order and ways to move around each other.
- Using their bodies, have them try it a second time and see how few passes they can do it in.

Items Needed:

different sized balls
racquets
bats
cardboard tubes
wood, etc.

Group Size:

2 or more

Format:

Pairs

Group

Group vs. Group

THE SEATED CHICKEN

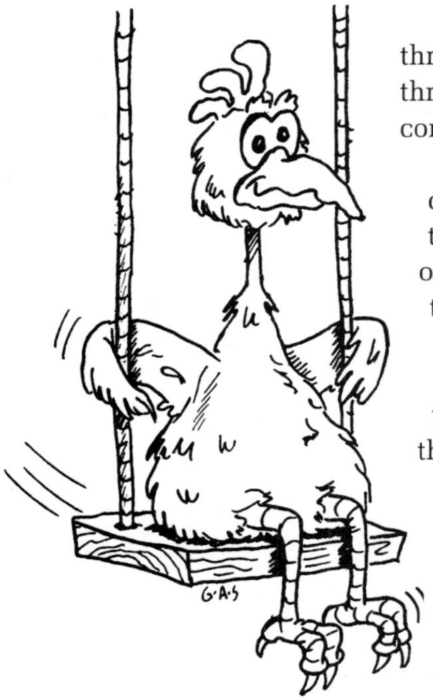

Everyone knows that every chicken must have a throne. The problem is that in these here parts, the only throne we have is a swing. That's where the group's help comes in.

The object of *The Seated Chicken* is to get a rubber chicken to stay seated, while it is swinging, by using only the items given. See *Junkyard Swing* for the basic set-up of *The Seated Chicken.* The wood does not need to swing the whole time, just as a test at the end when the group feels they have safely and securely seated the chicken.

Just as a point of clarification (because it *will* come up), the chicken may not be laying down or leaning over so that its chest hits its legs. As in *Fowl Play*, the chicken must be treated with the utmost respect at all times.

Procedure

Give them a short piece of string (about enough to make it around the wood twice and be knotted), two pieces of paper, a pencil and a rubber band to work with. They need not all be used. They may do whatever they want to their supplies, but they cannot get new ones. So if they cut the paper and then decide they want a whole sheet, they are out of luck. As in *Junkyard Swing,* the rope supports may not be used.

You don't have to use a rubber chicken if you don't have one. In fact, a floppy type of doll like a Raggedy Ann or a Sesame Street doll (we have used Elmo, for somewhat obvious reasons) will give a little extra support. Dolls with rigid backs, like traditional plastic dolls, make it significantly easier. Too easy, in fact, for most groups.

If they finish quickly, challenge them to come up with another way of solving it. If they finish this second attempt quickly, try it with new props.

When you are processing the experience, encourage clients to talk about their divergent thinking, full group involvement, and communication.

Items needed:

rubber chicken or flexible stuffed animal
2 foot long 2"x4" board
two, 3-foot lengths of rope
string
two pieces of paper
pencil
rubber band
2 chairs

Group Size: **2 or more**

Format: **Group**

SHOULDER TOSS

Shoulder Toss addresses primarily physical goals, but with minor modifications you can increase the cognitive and communicative demands. The props are velcro balls, the size of tennis balls; string, rubber bands or elastic (long enough to be tied around a waist; and 3 inch by 3 inch pieces of felt or velcro (depending on which type of velcro balls you have). The velcro balls are inexpensive and easy to find in most stores that sell toys. The object is to pass a velcro ball through the group via pieces of felt located on various body parts.

Variation I

Each person straps a piece of felt to his/her shoulder using a piece of string or elastic or a rubber band. Elastic and rubber bands work the best because they slide the least. The members must pass the ball around from shoulder to shoulder so that everyone has touched it. Like in *Warp Speed* (see *Cowstails and Cobras II,* p. 83), you can have the group see how fast they can pass it, doing it over and over until they don't think they could possibly do it a second faster.

Variation II

Everyone chooses two places on their body to put the pieces of felt. Have clients choose these two places before you tell them what they'll be doing. Discourage the group from putting the felt on their palms — too easy! They need to pass the ball from one part of their own body to the next *before* passing to the next person. They should try to anticipate which spot on their body is best to receive from, given the part of the body the person before them is passing from. For example, if the person before you has the ball on his shoulder and you have a choice of receiving it on your elbow or your foot, it would be better to receive it on your elbow. Of course, you would also have to consider where the felt is on the person you will be passing to!

After this round, some people may have discovered that it is physically impossible for them to pass from the one part of their body to the next. For example, it would be extremely hard, if not downright impossible to pass the ball to yourself from one shoulder to the other. If this is the case, allow those people to choose two new places and continue. The members can keep these felt positions in subsequent rounds and see how fast they can pass the ball, they can change these spots and keep passing, or they can pass to a new person each time.

Variation III

In another variation on this theme, they can pass to someone else before receiving it back to their second felt position. They have to remember who has had the ball and how many times.

Variation IV

Add more balls and watch the demands on information processing increase! Let them have some real fun and start the multiple balls going in opposite directions!

Each individual variation has the potential to be quick, so move from one to another, constantly changing the action as needed.

Debriefing

Discussion topics might include: physical compensations needed, comfort level with close contact with others, communication, planning, information processing speed or physical speed with multiple balls, and ease of one variation versus another.

Items needed: **velcro balls**
string, rubber bands, or elastic
felt

Group Size: **4 or more**

Format: **Group**

STAR TWIST

As you're walking down the hallway with the rope over your shoulder and the group following nervously behind you saying, "Oh no, not another rope thing," have some fun with them. Say something like, "Yeah, and this one could get messy. Are you ready for it?" Ask what they think this one will be like. Get some ideas flowing. Keep them talking until you have everyone gathered around you in an open area. Then get them started.

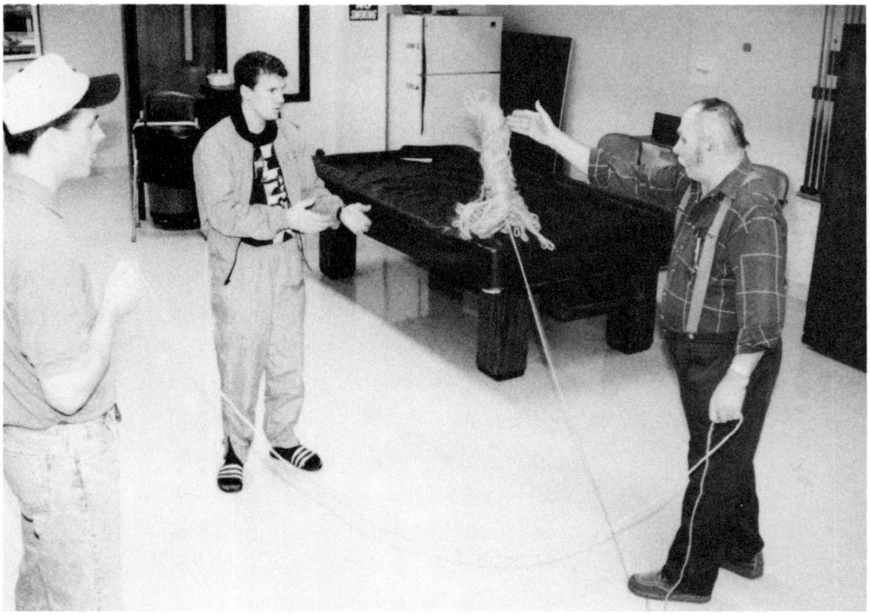

Procedure

Let the group know they'll be working on problem-solving and communication. Their goal in *Star Twist* is to form a five-point star with a rope. In the end of the activity, everyone must be touching the rope. One challenge for them will be how to form a five-point star with more than five people. When they decide they are ready to go for it, the group must take up their positions in a circle with a diameter of about ten feet. At this point, only one person may be holding the rope.

The first time, allow the rope to be thrown across the circle if the clients choose. The second time, though, change their positions around the circle and don't allow the rope to be tossed more than one foot. This will force them to change their strategy a bit. Have the group form other shapes if you like.

Blindfolding would be fun on this one, don't you think?

Items needed: **50-foot rope**

Group Size: **5 or more**

Format: **Group**

THE TRAVELER

The Traveler is a great activity for getting everyone up and moving about. It works on a variety of skills, including planning, communication, coordination and balance. The modes of travel listed below could be easily changed to accommodate more gross motor and high level balance goals.

Procedure

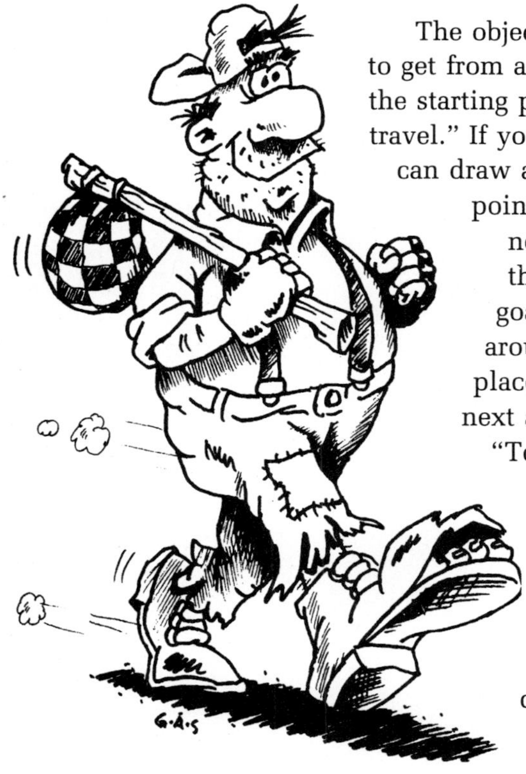

The object of *The Traveler* is for a team working together to get from a starting point to various other sites and back to the starting point, having used several specified "modes of travel." If you have enough time before the group starts, you can draw a map for them to follow. At each stopping point on the map, they pick up a card with their next mode of travel on it. Or, five minutes before the group starts, or as one leader is going over goal sheets with the group, the other leader can go around to each stop and tape a card in an obvious place. This card should have on it where they go next and how they should get there. For example: "To the lunch room moving as a triangle." In each mode of travel the entire group is working and moving together. So, in the above situation, the whole group needs to form a triangle and keep that shape until they have successfully made it to the lunch room. Some of the modes are easy and some require a bit of communication and reasoning. Try these modes and add your own.

Modes of Travel

- As a triangle, square, etc.
- Half face forward, half face backward
- Straight line, one behind the other, every other person facing backwards
- In pairs, back to back
- In a line, the sides of your feet touching the sides of the person's feet next to you. Your feet must remain touching the person's on your right and left the whole time you are traveling. This mode is very difficult to plan and execute if done correctly.
- Tapping your own head with one hand and tapping the shoulder of the person to your right with your other hand. (You may need to help clients compensate for upper extremity limits in range of motion or let them figure it out on their own.)
- Paired trust walk — one member with eyes closed, the other one telling him where to walk. The leaders typically act as moving obstacles here!
- March single file in order of middle name or last name, birth date, etc.
- Single file by height, whistling.

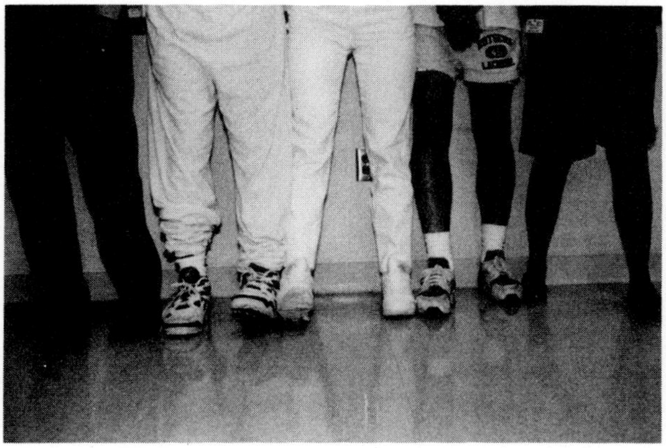

You only need to take the time to draw your map or write your cards once and then you should be ready to go each time you do *The Traveler* after that.

When you debrief, discuss how they were able to coordinate the whole group's actions, what was the easiest or hardest mode of travel and why, and how they compensated for physical deficits.

Items needed: **index cards with locations and modes of travel on them**

Group Size: **4 or more**

Format: **Group**

WALKIE TALKIE TOWERS

This one is difficult. It's a variation of the classic barrier communication activities. The heaviest demand is on communication, specifically precision in direction giving and asking questions. If you haven't guessed already, the difficult (and frustrating) part is the barrier. You can't see what's happening on the other side of it. You can't even see if they have heard you.

Procedure

The group is divided into two teams and set up in two different rooms. Each team is given a walkie talkie. One group creates something with materials given and must tell the other group, via the walkie talkie, how to create the exact same thing. For our materials, we like to use large, various sized and shaped pieces of wood so clients get their whole body involved lifting and hauling the materials. Large objects also increase the potential need for group cooperation. But you can use blocks, paper or anything else you've got hanging around instead, as long as you have two identical sets.

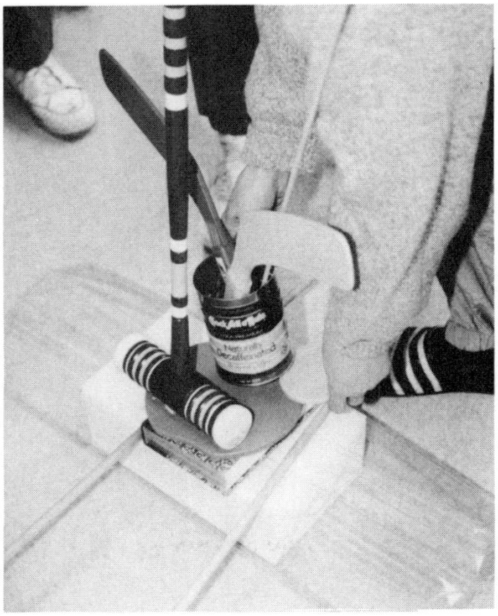

The responsibility for success is placed on both groups — one must give the directions clearly, but the other must ask for clarification. You can make this point up front in the brief or maybe talk about it later during the debrief. Putting the responsibility on both groups encourages more question asking and eliminates blaming when the end products don't match. If time allows, let both groups have an opportunity to be on each side of the direction giving.

Modifications

In nice weather, you can use two different sides of the building, or, when your batteries have died (or if you don't even have walkie talkies), you can use a room divider, a curtain, a door, or anything else you can think of.

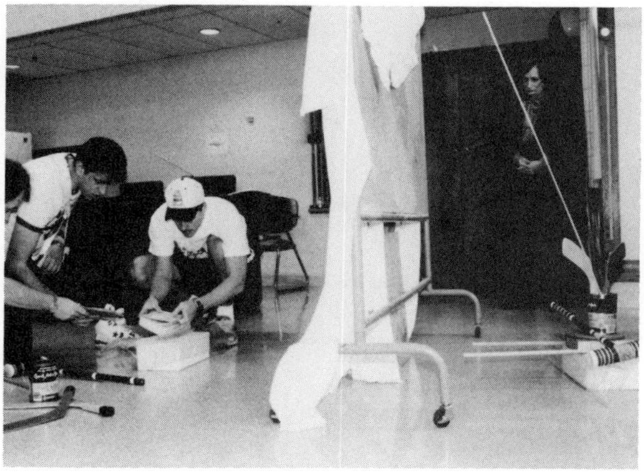

Items needed: **various sized and shaped pieces of wood (2 of each)**
blocks or other miscellaneous stuff (2 of each)
walkie talkies (optional)
some type of divider (wall, door, curtain, rolling blackboard, etc.)

Group Size: **2 or more**

Format: **Group vs. Group**
Pairs

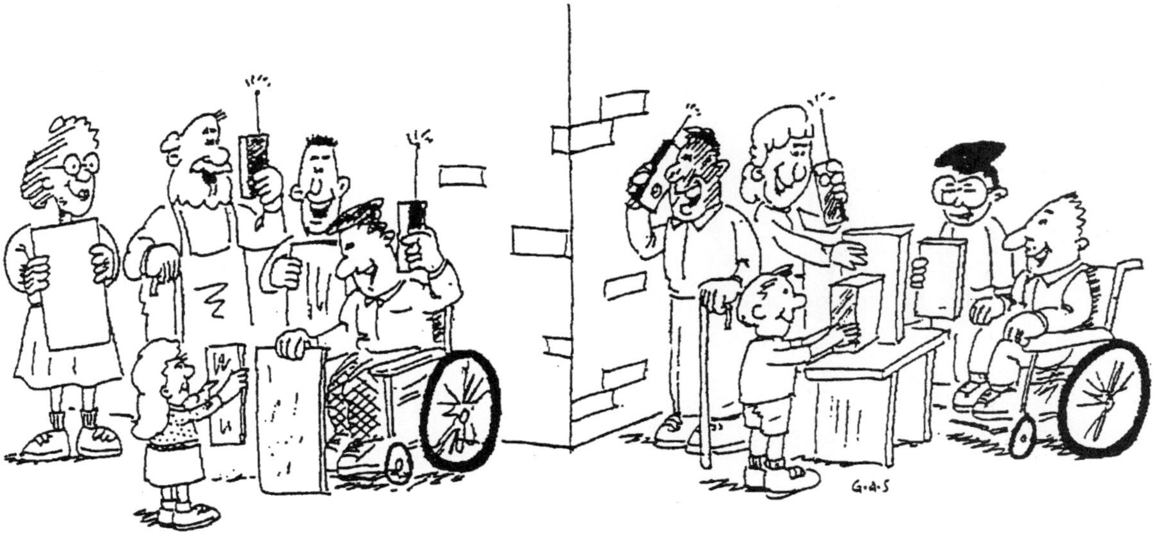

WALL WALKERS
(Or SCALE THE WALL II)

In this version of *Scale the Wall,* the ball travels along the wall through an obstacle course. This is a good version to use if you are working with shorter people (kids) or people in wheelchairs. You can use any of the modifications from *Scale the Wall* that you like: for instance, props or bodies, groups or pairs, etc. The same rules apply as in *Wall Walkers* for dropping or catching a ball.

The *Wall Walkers* obstacle course can be set up in a number of different ways. You can have them:

- Weave around things that are already on the wall like pictures, outlets, windows.
- Follow a map.
- Follow the verbal directions of a teammate. The direction followers can be blindfolded or not.
- Go through pipe cleaner underpasses (like in croquet). The real word for those things escapes us. You will probably have to use golf ball-sized balls.
- Follow masking tape arrows. If you choose this option, please use a brick wall so that you do not get fired for taking all the paint off the walls when you remove the tape.

Items needed:

balls
racquets, bats or cardboard tubes
other items needed depend on how you make your obstacle course — see above for ideas

Group Size: **2 or more**

Format:

Group
Group vs. Group
Pairs

WETDOWN

Wetdown is best played outdoors for soon-to-be-obvious reasons. It is nice on a warm day when the threat of getting wet would actually be welcomed. Most of our clients get nervous when they see the water balloons in *Wetdown*. It might have something to do with long suppressed memories of running away from older brothers while screaming, "Don't throw it! Don't throw it! Maaa!" And then hearing a splat and feeling cold wetness as your shirt sticks to your back. Really, though, their fears are unwarranted. The most wet that clients ever get is a few splattered drops on their shins from a water balloon that dropped at their feet.

Procedure

The main props are water balloons and lunch trays (or wood or hard cardboard, etc.). The group is divided into two teams and then each team is broken down into couples. One couple from each team approaches the starting line and is given a tray to hold wrong side up, horizontally between them. A water balloon is placed on each tray. They must race the other couple to the end line 15–20 feet away, without letting their water balloon drop. At the end, they put the balloon in a bucket and the next couple from their team goes. Technically, the team with the most balloons in their bucket wins, but we usually end up grabbing balloons from the buckets prematurely to replace ones that have fallen off the trays and become casualties of fun. This makes for a non-competitive, just-have-fun atmosphere.

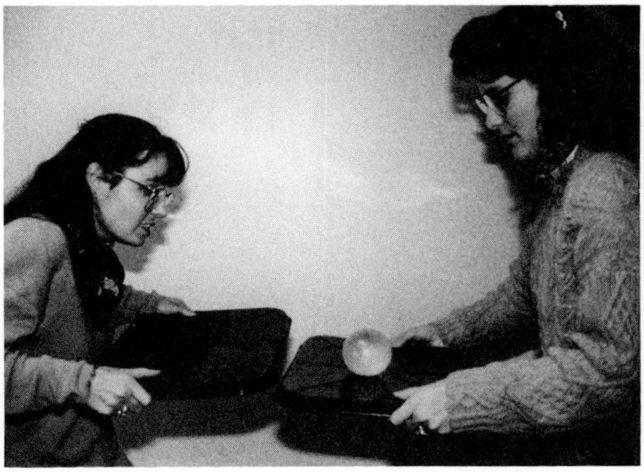

Wheelchair users can participate in *Wetdown* and we have had success including people with use of only one arm, too.

Debriefing

When you process the *Wetdown* experience with the group, you might discuss what they needed in order to balance the balloon on the tray — attention, physical coordination, communication with their partner. You may have noted that there wasn't always a lot of talking between the partners, yet they were still effective. Why was this?

Variations

Once they have made a couple of attempts doing it "successfully" with one balloon, we add a second. We have only had a very few couples who have made it from start to finish without dropping at least one balloon. Next, *all* of the couples are given trays and the balloons must be passed from one couple's tray to the next in line. It's hard, try it! The variations are really limitless. You could work up to an obstacle course or use different objects on the trays.

One caution — be sure to wipe wet feet before coming back inside to highly buffed floors!

Items needed:
20 water balloons
lunch trays or wood squares
2 buckets

Group Size: **4 or more**

Format: **Pairs**
Group vs. Group

WHICH WAY DID THEY GO?

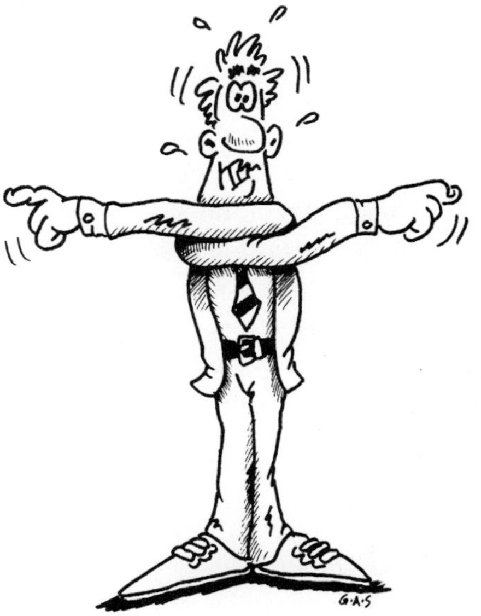

Which Way Did They Go? is good for groups that do not require a lot of structure. It would be best if this one was done some time after a clue hunt because they will have to develop some clues of their own. Having previously done a clue hunt will give clients some frame of reference to go by.

Procedure

Divide the group into two teams and assign each a mascot. These mascots should be hidden in different places by the therapists before the session starts. Tell each team where the other's mascot is. Each group must develop and then leave clues for the other team leading them to their mascot. They should be encouraged to leave different types of clues — written, visual, etc. Each clue should lead to the next one. Specify a certain number of clues to be left. They need to be careful while they are out placing their clues because the other team will be out placing theirs, as well. They don't want to be seen.

When both groups are done placing their clues, they can go in search of the other team's mascot by looking for their clues. All of the clues must be found in order to be considered successful.

Some groups may need reminding that the clues need to be reasonable. They should not be so farfetched, unreasonable or hidden that the other group will not be able to find them. Remind clients that their goal is to enable the other group to find the mascot, but also to make them think in the process.

Debriefing

There will probably be a lot of content for the debrief. Allow the groups time to give each other feedback about the clues the other team developed for them. They can discuss what was more difficult — creating or solving clues. Ask clients what skills they used. They might list: planning, logical thinking, communication and maybe creativity.

Items needed: **2 odd objects**

Group Size: **4 or more**

Format: **Pairs**
Group vs. Group

WHO'S DRIVING THAT CAR?

With *Who's Driving That Car?,* we begin by telling the group that we were out driving around yesterday and saw some license plates that gave a clue to the drivers' occupations. We want their help in figuring out what job they might do. They need to list as many jobs as they can that might apply.

Procedure

You can introduce more competition by dividing the group in half and having them compete against each other. When they are done (or the time limit has expired), bring the groups back together to share their answers. Every answer common to both groups should be crossed off so that, in the end, only unique answers remain. The group with the most remaining occupations wins. This process of going through and discussing answers will take awhile, so don't just allow the normal amount of debriefing time. In a 45-minute session, you might allow 5 minutes to brief and go over goals, 15 minutes to come up with their answers, 15 minutes to go over them and 10 minutes to debrief and fill out goal sheets. If you like, you could allow one session to come up with answers and a second session to go over them.

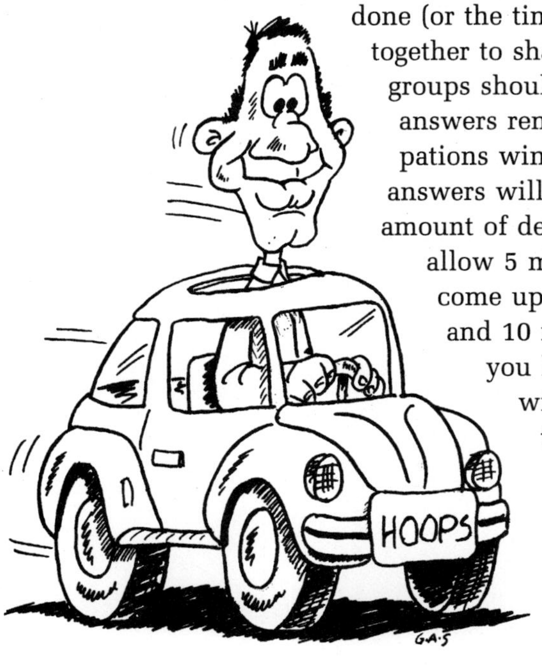

Encourage clients to challenge their divergent thinking skills and let their creative juices flow. As long as they can defend their answers and the majority agrees, the answers will be counted. The group leaders should vote as well.

Debriefing

In the end, discuss divergent thinking and word-finding. People with word-finding difficulties may find *Who's Driving That Car?* a real challenge. But maybe their role can be describing an occupation sufficiently to enable their teammates to guess what they're thinking of. Then the role of teamwork would be a great topic to discuss. Another typically relevant topic would be their approach. Did they pick one license plate and stick with it to exhaust all possibilities and not leave enough time to get to all of them? Or did they spend a few minutes on each one and maybe only come up with a few answers?

Suggestions:

ACE	SMILE	MOWMAN
NAILS	BOOKER	BONES
WORDS	COLLECTOR	TUNEMAKER
MR FOOD	MONEYMN	ROCKY
BUZZ	MR SUDZ	HOOPS
SMELLY	SPARKY	FLY ME
TOP GUN	TOP DOG	SHARK

Items Needed: **license plates listed on paper with spaces for answers**

Group Size: **4 or more**

Format: **Group vs. Group**
Group
Pairs

Appendices

Appendix I

Activities By Group Size

Keep in mind that this appendix, in the case of most activities, should serve as a general guide. There is room for lots of flexibility. The numbers represent a *minimum* number needed. So, if you have eight people, all of the activities are potentially good for your group's size. Some are inherently more suited for less people and some for more people. When choosing an activity according to group size, also remember that one or both group leaders may also participate, unless they are needed for spotting.

1 or more

Gamemaster

2 or more

Get Outa Town
No Sneezing
Pile-on
Alien Invasion
Scale the Wall
Wall Walkers
Balloom
Junkyard Swing
The Seated Chicken
Chain Reaction
Decode the Code
Fillet of Sole
Pack Your Bags
Walkie Talkie Towers

3 or more

Get it Together
The Name Game
Road Trip
Rocky Road
Get it Straight
Move it or Lose it

4 or more

All Tied Up
Blind Spear Fishing
Bullseye
Bullseye II
Burglars and Lasers
Chutes and 'Loons
Cobweb
Crossword
Dressing Relay
Is It?
Lost Your Marbles
Mystery Clue Hunt
Orb Escape
Pile-on Competition
Sacred Chalice Rescue
Shoulder Toss
The Traveler
Wetdown
Who's Driving That Car
The Pit
Fowl Play
Which Way Did They Go
Bend, Bump and Roll
Get it Straight

5 or more

One Lump or Two?
Star Twist

6 or more

Drawing Relay
Passing Lane
Body Building

Appendix II

Activities By Format

Many of the activities are repeated under more than one format because they are flexible.

Group

Passing Lane
One Lump or Two
The Seated Chicken
Junkyard Swing
Fowl Play
Balloom
Wall Walkers
Scale the Wall
All Tied Up
Cobweb
Crossword
Decode the Code
Fillet of Sole
Gamemaster
Get it Straight
Get Outa Town
Move it or Lose it
The Name Game
No Sneezing
Orb Escape
Pack Your Bags
Pile-on
Road Trip
Sacred Chalice Rescue
Shoulder Toss
The Traveler
Who's Driving That Car
Rocky Road
Chain Reaction
Alien Invasion
Star Twist
Get it Together
Mystery Clue Hunt
Pile-on Competition

Pairs

Blind Spear Fishing
Bullseye
Bullseye II
Burglars and Lasers
Chutes and 'Loons
Crossword
Dressing Relay
Bend, Bump and Roll
Lost Your Marbles
Mystery Clue Hunt
No Sneezing
Pile-on Competition
Walkie Talkie Towers
Wetdown
Who's Driving That Car
The Pit
Scale the Wall
Wall Walkers
Which Way Did They Go

Group vs. Group

Chutes and 'Loons
Crossword
Drawing Relay
Is It?
Mystery Clue Hunt
No Sneezing
Pile-on Competition
Road Trip
Walkie Talkie Towers
Wetdown
Who's Driving That Car
The Pit
Scale the Wall
Wall Walkers
Body Building
Which Way Did They Go
Bend, Bump and Roll

Appendix III

Activities: Table Top Versus Up and Moving

Appendix IV should serve as a quick guide when you need to shift gears from outside to inside because of weather, when you need to vary the intensity because of a missing co-leader, or when you just want to give the group some variety.

Table Top

Crossword
Decode the Code
Fillet of Sole
Gamemaster
Get it Together
Get Outa Town
The Name Game
Pack Your Bags
Pile-on
Road Trip
Who's Driving That Car?
Is it?
Lost Your Marbles
Pile-on Competition
Chain Reaction
Bend, Bump and Roll
Drawing Relay
No Sneezing

Up and Moving

All Tied Up
Cobweb
Get it Straight
Move it or Lose it
No Sneezing
Orb Escape
Sacred Chalice Rescue
The Traveler
Blind Spear Fishing
Bullseye
Bullseye II
Burglars and Lasers
Chutes and 'Loons
Dressing Relay
Mystery Clue Hunt
Walkie Talkie Towers
Wetdown
Drawing Relay
The Pit
Rocky Road
Alien Invasion
Scale the Wall
Wall Walkers
Balloom
Fowl Play
Junkyard Swing
The Seated Chicken
One Lump or Two
Passing Lane
Star Twist
Body Building
Which Way Did They Go?
Shoulder Toss

Appendix IV

Activities From Other Sources

Source: ***Silver Bullets***

by Karl Rohnke, Project Adventure, Inc. 1984

Activity	**Page #**
Toss-A-Name Game	pg. 17 — Add variation of "tossing" goals.
Minefield	pg. 24 — Use common objects from other activities, allow person giving directions to stand next his partner; wheelchairs and walkers may touch objects but people cannot.
Paper Golf	pg. 33
Which Way? Softball	pg. 34 — Play on paper instead of on softball diamond.
Impulse	pg. 35
Hands Down	pg. 53
Passing Crossed or Uncrossed	pg. 55
I've Got the Beat	pg. 55
Circle the Circle	pg. 60 — Not good for wheelchairs or walkers.
Hoop Relay	pg. 61 — Not for walkers or wheelchairs.
Bump	pg. 68

Activity	Page #
Trust Fall	pg. 80 — We do only a trust lean.
Wordles	pg. 103
TP Shuffle	pg. 110 — Our "log" is actually tape on the floor.
Group Juggling	pg. 112
Knots	pg. 117-118
Macro Tangrams	pg. 129
Trolley	pg. 118-119 — Not for wheelchairs or walkers.
2 x 4	pg. 123 — We allow our groups to solve it first with paper cups because it is too difficult for them to do it with people only.
The Almost Infinite Circle	pg. 131

Source: ***Cowstails and Cobras II***

by Karl Rohnke, Project Adventure, Inc., 1989

Activity	Page #
What Goes Where?	pg. 65
Hustle Handle	pg. 66
Yurt Circle	pg. 73 — Beware of decreased range of motion or weakness in upper extremities.
Blind Polygon, Blindfold Square	pg. 81
The Meuse	pg. 82 — We keep things low to the ground by having them walk across paneling.

Activity	Page #
Warp Speed	pg. 83
The Great Egg Drop	pg. 85-86
Object Retrieval	pg. 86 — In our variation, they rescue a basket from the middle of the circle using only the props given. We do not allow them to extend any part of their bodies across the "pit" area. If they do, they lose the ability to use that part of their bodies for the remain der of the activity.
The Maze	pg. 104

Source: ***More New Games***

The New Games Foundation, 1981

Activity	Page #
Me Switch	pg. 19
Quick Draw	pg. 21
This is My Nose	pg. 27
Willow in the Wind	pg. 67
Instant Replay	pg. 71
A What?	pg. 73
Zen Clap	pg. 79
Elephant/Palm Tree/Monkey	pg. 147

Source: ***Bottomless Baggie***

by Karl Rohnke, Kendall/Hunt Publishing Co., 1991

Activity	**Page #**
Knee Slap	pg. 1
Silly Veggies	pg. 10
Acronyms and Initialisms	pg. 16
Just Lying Around	pg. 26
I'm Thumbody	pg. 26
Grid Code	pg. 31
The Square Route	pg. 34
Roller Ball	pg. 45
Buddy Ropes	pg. 46
Listening Skills	pg. 47
Junkyard Traverse	pg. 49
3D Minefield	pg. 50
Wordles	pg. 86

Games Index

Project Adventure Services

Since 1971 Project Adventure has been creating learning programs that challenge people to go beyond their perceived boundaries, to work with others to solve problems and to experience success. Over 1 million people have used our approach to realize increased self-confidence, develop leadership skills, discover the power of group cooperation, and learn to view obstacles as opportunities for growth.

The Project Adventure concept is characterized by an atmosphere that is fun, supportive and challenging. Non-competitive games, group problem solving Initiatives and ropes course events are the principal activities we use to help individuals reach their goals; to improve self-esteem, to develop strategies that enhance decision-making, and to respect differences within a group.

We offer the following services:

Project Adventure Workshops

Through a network of national certified trainers, Project Adventure conducts workshops for teachers, counselors, youth workers and other professionals who work with people. These workshops are given in various sections of the country. Separate workshops are given in Challenge Ropes Course Skills, Counseling Skills for Adventure Based Programs, Project Adventure Games and Initiatives, and Interdisciplinary Academic Curriculum.

Program Accreditation

The Accreditation process is an outside review of a program by PA staff. Programs that undertake the accreditation process are seeking outside evaluation with regard to quality and safety. The term accreditation means "formal written confirmation." Programs seeking confirmation are looking to ensure that they are within the current standards of safety and risk management. This assurance may be useful for making changes in program equipment and/or design, and in providing information on program quality to third parties such as administrators, insurance companies and the public.

Challenge Course Equipment Catalog

A catalog service of hard-to-find materials and tools used in the installation of Challenge Ropes Courses. This catalog also contains climbing rope and a variety of items useful to adventure programs.

Challenge Course Design and Installation

Project Adventure has been designing and installing ropes courses (a series of individual and group challenge elements situated indoors in a gymnasium or outdoors in a grove of trees) for over 15 years. PA Staff can travel to your site and design/install a course appropriate for your needs and budget.

Professional Development

Management workshops for business and professional persons. These workshops are designed for increasing efficiency of team members in the workplace. The trust, communication, and risk-taking ability learned in the executive programs translate into a more cohesive and productive team at work.

Program Accreditation.

The Accreditation process is an outside review of a program by PA staff. Programs that undertake the accreditation process are seeking outside evaluation with regard to quality and safety. The term accreditation means "formal written confirmation." Programs seeking confirmation are looking to ensure that they are within the current standards of safety and risk management. This assurance may be useful for making changes in program equipment and/or design, and in providing information on program quality to third parties such as administrators, insurance companies and the public.

Publications

Project Adventure, Inc. publishes books and other material for the field of Experiential and Adventure Education. Our titles cover such diverse subjects as: games, Initiatives and Adventure activities, theory, leadership, and safety. An order form is provided on the next page that includes some our best sellers, which are described below. Call or write Project Adventure for a compete publications list.

Cowstails and Cobras II

The 1989 revision of Karl Rohnke's classic guide to games, Initiatives, and Adventure and trust activities contains much of what made the original a classic in the field. This expanded edition includes sections on leadership issues and curriculum outlines from model programs.

SilverBullets

More Initiative problems, Adventure games and trust activities from Karl Rohnke: 165 great games and activities that require few, if any, props. Use this as a companion to *Cowstails and Cobras II* or a stand alone guide to invigorate your program.

Islands Of Healing

Subtitled *A Guide to Adventure Based Counseling, Islands* presents a comprehensive discussion of this rapidly growing counseling approach. Started in 1974, ABC is an innovative, group counseling model that uses cooperative games, Initiative problem solving, low and high Challenge Ropes Course elements, and other Adventure activities. The book contains extensive "how-to" information on group selection, training, goal setting, sequencing, and leading and debriefing activities. Also included are explorations of model ABC programs at several representative sites — junior and senior high schools, a psychiatric hospital, and court referred programs. By Jim Schoel, Dick Prouty, and Paul Radcliffe.

SilverBullets Video

This first of its kind video presents Karl leading 20 of the best Project Adventure games and Initiatives. The video guides viewers through the events as Karl presents instructions, variations, safety tips, unique ways to choose sides, implementation help, and insights that come from doing these events for 20 years. The video goes beyond what the books can do because you actually see the games played out — from beginning to often riotous end. Also included is a field manual that outlines rules, goals, safety considerations and leadership issues that present different perspectives to each event. *Running time: 2:05*

Adventure Based Counseling Videos

On of the basic tenets of experiential education holds that we learn best by doing. But if we can't always be immersed in the doing atmosphere of a workshop, then perhaps the next best thing is to watch others doing. These two videos offer just that — a unique chance to see many of the concepts of Adventure Based Counseling and *Islands Of Healing* in action. The videos simulate an Adventure Based Counseling program within an institutional setting. Both videos are appropriate for either ongoing or one-day programs.

Video One demonstrates such concepts as Challenge By Choice and the Full Value Contract by portraying actual activities — *Balloon Frantic, Willow in the Wind* and *Mine Field.* Several debriefing techniques are also presented, such as go 'round and what-so what-now what. *Running Time — 43:00*

Video Two focuses on the Adventure Wave by presenting three activities — *Flip Me the Bird Tag, Wild Woosey* and *Prouty's Landing* and highlighting briefing, leading and debriefing techniques. *Running Time — 38:00*

Office Locations

Project Adventure has four offices in the U.S. and overseas in Canada, Singapore, Australia and New Zealand. You can get information by writing or calling any of the offices listed below. Book orders should be sent to one of the addresses listed at the bottom of the order form.

Project Adventure, Inc

P.O. Box 100
Hamilton, MA 01936
508/468-7981
FAX 508/468-7605

P.O. Box 2447
Covington, GA 30209
404/784-9310
FAX 404/787-7764

116 Maple St,
Brattleboro, VT 05301
802/254-5054
FAX 802/254-5182

P.O. Box 14171
Portland, OR 97214
503/239-0169
FAX 503/236-6765

Order/Request Form

Please send information on the following:

- ❑ **Project Adventure Training Workshops**
- ❑ **Challenge Course Design and Installation**
- ❑ **Ropes Course Equipment Catalog**
- ❑ **Executive Reach Programs**
- ❑ **Publications List**
- ❑ **Program Accreditation**
- ❑ **Please add my name to your mailing list**

Qty	Title	Price	Total
	Cowstails and Cobras II	18.50	
	Silver Bullets	18.50	
	Islands of Healing	20.50	
	ABC Video One	45.00	
	ABC Video Two	45.00	
	Silver Bullets Video	45.95	
	Adapted Adventure	19.50	

Subtotal ________

5% tax (Mass. residents only) ________

Shipping (instructions below) ________

TOTAL ________

Shipping Instructions

Orders up to $35.00 — add $3.50
Orders over $35.00 — add 10% of total
(Canada & overseas, add additional $2.00 to total)

Ship to:

Name ________

Address ________

City ________ State ________ Zip ________

Phone (____) ________

Payment:

❑ Check enclosed ❑ Purchase Order

Charge to: ❑ Visa ❑ MasterCard

Card # ________ Exp. ________

Signature ________

(Signature required for all charge orders.)

Copy or detach this form and return to:

Project Adventure, Inc.
P.O. Box 100
Hamilton, MA 01936
508/468-7981
FAX: 508/468-7605

or

P.O. Box 2447
Covington, GA 30209
404/784-9310
FAX: 404/787-7764